NEUROPHILOSOPHY OF CONSCIOUSNESS, VOL. VII

THE UNEXPECTED TRANSITION FROM IDEALISM TO REALISM

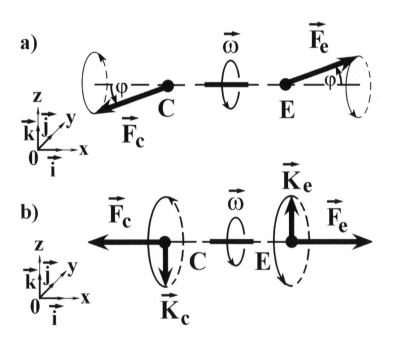

Dr. Angell O. de la Sierra, Esq.

An Update on Dirac's Transactional Interpretation Quantum Mechanics Model (TIQM) as modified for a BioPsychoSocial (BPS) Model of Human Brain Dynamics.

Order this book online at www.trafford.com
or email orders@trafford.com

Most Trafford titles are also available at major online book retailers.

Printed in the United States of America.

ISBN: 978-1-4907-1238-3 (sc)
ISBN: 978-1-4907-1237-6 (e)

Trafford rev. 09/09/2013

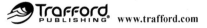

www.trafford.com

North America & international
toll-free: 1 888 232 4444 (USA & Canada)
fax: 812 355 4082

CONTENTS

INTRODUCTION

General. There should really be nothing tricky or mysterious about faith values, whether the reference frame belief is theosophist, atheist, scientologist, agnostic or their variations. In normal, healthy human beings all beliefs have a common denominator, either they are rooted on sensory (phenomenological) factual observations, measurements of physical objects or events or rooted on extrasensory (non-phenomenological logical probabilities that can be inferred from those descriptions) explanations. The credibility of any ensuing judgment depends on the falsifiable consistence and predictability of the occurrence in question under standard environmental conditions during a given moment in time and space location. Another important aspect of the credibility of a given judgment is related to the probable truth content of either the sensory experience (ontology) or the extrasensory logical inference (epistemology) directly relevant to the occurrence being analyzed for reliable truth content.

It should be obvious that the sensory ontological/physical presence is directly verifiable whereas the extrasensory epistemological/metaphysical 'presence' is based on their probability of occurrence. Please consider that the object or event may be physically present but outside the threshold of the human brain sensory resolution (such as microorganisms, molecules, atoms, etc.). In this case its physical but invisible presence has to be established inferentially by the predictable consequences of its probable presence if and only we can justify with logical arguments a probable direct causally efficient agency responsible for the predictable consequences epistemologically. In the absence of direct sensory information we now properly substitute the perceptual information with temporary, reliable cognitive information, the epistemological inference. Hopefully in the future a positive prediction of the occurrence is reinforced by instrumental micro descriptions of the direct causally efficient physical agents. It is also possible to infer a probable physical causal agency by functional criteria based on their predictable influence on specific brain loci activity as indirectly measured by falsifiable f-MRI recordings. Notice how we depart from a direct sensory experience to an indirect instrumental equivalent. Can this equivalence still reside inside the ontological domain of discourse, quare.

But, what if a direct or indirect physical causal agent may not even be ontologically described or epistemologically explained?

Specific. Enter the domain of the hybrid model-poem 'singularity' we have baptized as the 'Epistemontological' biopsychosocial (BPS) unit model of brain dynamics. We hope that by attempting (an unfinished work yet) a reconciliation and modification of the well documented and reliable ontological and epistemological literature it will provide another credible and truthful restatement of the age old question 'what is the absolute nature of human conscious existential reality'. In so doing it will add another dimension to the ongoing discourse on the evolution of complexity as it underscores the human species biopsychosocial survival imperative against natural destructive odds and the human exclusive capacity to transcend the primitive BPS mode to create the unique civilization no other advanced species can. The transcendental escape from the limiting 4-d space-time Minkowsky biosphere into transfinite manifolds is an ongoing effort to search for credible and convincing answers to explain the elusive conundrum of human life and consciousness that survives across generations while other better adapted species become history.

Unfortunately, many intelligent and well educated humans have not been able to escape and transcend the limiting scope of their exclusive BPS existential reality. Instead they use their natural intellectual endowments to pursue the self indulging conveniences of power, wealth and control, many a times at the expense of the less fortunate citizens that are entitled also to be healthy, happy and cooperatively convivial so they can actively participate in the creation of our progressive civilization to the extent of their endowed capacities. Consequently, there is no doubt about the biological survival priority of preserving all life, that is the proper role of organized religions in the Judeo ChrIslamic tradition and their equivalent belief systems whether atheistic, agnostic or scientological. Once the neuro-humoral control of the emotional aspects of ongoing existence, those that properly creates the psychosocial emotional experience of blind faith when exposed to it, it now needs to add another dimension of belief for those with those interests, commitments, curiosity and abilities to carry them on as documented in recorded history accounts as the life of the prophets. These prophets and their equivalents are the few ones that have carried the burden of preserving human lives against the evolving unfavorable odds across generations.

What institutions will produce the new prophets of the 21st. Century, the materialist cults, the radical extreme religionists, the Sartrean hedonic existentialists or the updated religious institutions? The update consists in providing additional rational arguments for those already enjoying the emotional faith to consolidate their belief. We have seen how as the result of the technological information explosion new generations have evolved free from the shackles of radical extremists in the Middle East and in our local midst. In a more sophisticated way the technological information explosion has also generated the means of creating controls, greed, wealth and power for exploitation of the 'condemned of the earth' as we witness the globalization of the economy and the monopolistic capitalism effort to control the means of production at the expense of others less fortunate in resources to survive the new technology demands, a new version of 'survival of the fittest' at any cost and it may worsen as the traditional religious organizations continue their radical rituals ignoring the societal unrelenting evolutionary paths towards an exclusive radical materialistic interpretation of reality fueled by the information explosion. Reasonable human beings are caught in the middle of two extremes. Adherents of the materialist physicalist cults are now geared to grab attention and power using epistemological tools and unconvincing arguments suggesting that theoretical constructs of reality can create reality. Like suggesting that predicates or attributes of objects/events like their shape, form or color can exist independently from the object/event that made it possible! The map abstract virtual representation created the 'real' phenomenological territory being mapped!

I think the confusion with epistemology is that many a times it is the result of a deliberate attempt by some scholars to market their ideas with no concern for their probable truth content, so long as their ideas' sales pitch look brainy and elegant; it's mostly about low brow human self-indulgence. If everybody, anywhere, always, in a predictable and consistent way gets sick with same signs and symptoms because of their traceable <u>common</u> denominator experience of e.g., eating dirty fruits or never washing their hands when eating, then it is not necessary to always insist on the healer to demonstrate a sensory-based phenomenological identity of the specific offending bacteria/microorganism to relieve a patient of his acute ailment. One can cognitively posit the presence of offending microorganisms invisible to the naked eye when based on the epistemological knowledge of the consistent and predictable consequences of their environmental physical presence. This is the easiest scenario for illustration purposes of how always ignoring other complex etiological probable causal agents may bring future problems.

The confusion arises when dealing with very complex events dynamically evolving. In this scenario the indirect knowledge of a causally efficient agency may properly substitute the acute factual, phenomenological agent perceptual identification phase until the latter can at least be temporarily inferred as probable in a later future chronic phase evolution from the obvious observable consequences it causes in the present.

The confusion is at times compounded by the 'expert' practitioners when the predicate virtual consequences become 'animated' by their users and are made to become a magical mysterious reality independent from the 'real' physical causal agent that made it possible!!

Unfortunately there will always be consistently-experienced consequences that will escape sensory <u>description</u> or even <u>explanatory</u> epistemological inferences when linguistic precision is absent to infer a probable explanation. This last scenario is the fertile soil that breeds the model poems of reality appealing only to the emotional component of our existential reality that all religions properly encourage to keep people safely alive, feeling happy and socially/cooperatively convivial like we see our pets and zoo animals behaving like.

But we cannot leave out the rational component for the sake of completeness, we need to integrate both the physical ontological-perceptual description and the metaphysical epistemological-conceptualization of coexisting/interacting dynamic variables waiting for an adequate linguistic representation in symbolic or sentential logic format that facilitates their causally efficient analysis of probable etiology.

If we can distinguish the epistemological conceptual explanation from the ontological perceptual description of the same object/event and see the need to consider both as a complementary unit whole; the 'real' empirical with the 'ideal' probability, then it shouldn't be so difficult to understand the details of the complex argumentation that follows.

To better appreciate the overwhelming complexity of an objective analysis, it should be noticed the number and quality of the physical ontological **descriptions** of the object/event as perceptually sensed, measured or observed, directly or indirectly with instruments, from the derived metaphysical, epistemological conceptualizations **explanation**s directly or indirectly from such sense-phenomenal participating object or event. The conceptual representation may be expressed in symbolic or sentential logic for ease of analysis.

When engaged in the conceptualization effort we need also to distinguish the immediate invariant from the mediate variable parameters dynamically interacting or not. Dirac's <bra-ket> model genially conceptualized and we modified is a complete model of our 4-dimensional mesoscopic existential reality conceptualized as 9-dimensional virtual reality as published and briefly explained below. Equally relevant are clear distinctions between the inherited or acquired origin/source of the information content. As we discover more and more examples of microorganisms and chemicals ability to modify and causally influence the RNA transcription process of the inherited DNA the less importance we should give this blurred distinction between the inherited and the learned, the physically 'real' emotional experience and the 'ideal' virtual model of probable causality as metaphysically reasoned.

Last but not least in importance is the language syntax structure of the adopted language when reporting, in either subjective first or objective third person, a narrative model-poem account of the occurrence.

Almost exhaustive searches for the simplest analytical tool capable of generating a credible model poem encompassing all the identified relevant complex variables at play, suggested a new modified combination of Cramer's classic 'transactional model' and Dirac's original <bra-ket> notation analytical approach, all being published in numerous blogs and many book volumes sold by Amazon Books, Inc. including a "Treatise on Neurophilosophy of Consciousness, a BPS Model of Brain Dynamics" and 6 volumes of textbooks with similar titles. Most of this content can be found in our family domain site at <http://delaSierra-Sheffer. net> and a blog site at: <http://angelldls.wordpress.com/>.

We found it convenient to adopt and modify Dirac's model to account for the space-time evolutionary path of a dynamically evolving 'real' supercomplexity as brilliantly modeled in the original transactional interpretation of quantum mechanics (TIQM) 'ideal' virtual reality as we briefly discuss below under 'speculations and conjectures'.

Perhaps the most important feature of this model approach is the distinction between the **invariant** features of the 'ideal' **unit dimensional submicroscopic** physical particle component as they interactively aggregate into the 'real' eventual **total macroscopic** bulk with characteristic measurable identifying attributions we describe as their predicates. We will stress the importance of model virtual representations which must derive from solid falsifiable inputs of information as best illustrated by the 'twistor' theory. We need to focus more on the more complex virtual epistemological linguistic representation of the 'ideal' variable components of the complete 'Epistemontological' hybrid reality as monitored in the dynamic physical human brain. The ontological component is the measurable 'real' component we measure or observe in the laboratory. Together they form a complete model.

ARGUMENTATION

The Transactional Interpretation of Quantum Mechanics (TIQM) still faces a number of valid challenges. We will briefly address some of the fundamental criticisms mentioned in the Introduction above. According to the original account (See Cramer 1986), a transactional interpretation (TI) explains the 'ideal' transaction as a four-vector standing wave whose endpoints are the emission and absorption events. Its usefulness has been challenged on the basis of its actual 4-dimensional space-time process or is it just taking place on a level of possibility rather than a 'real' measurable actuality. We argue on the limited information processing resolution capacities of the human brain and thus the justification of the 'ideal' model is validated on its predictable 'real' phenomenal occurrences when ontologically confirmed, i.e., when the truth content of the putative 'ideal' indeterminate causal forces logically driving the occurrences as probable become determinate causal forces and more credible in 'real' mesoscopic life as measured in the brain dynamics laboratory.

In my opinion, many learned scientists and philosophers scholars have neglected to consider that either 'real' or 'ideal' interpretation is inevitably the account version of a human being linguistic narrative to other human beings with all the species cognitive and sensory limitations that it entails as briefly exposed below.

Mathematical justifications and precision. In my personal opinion the 'offer waves' (OW) fit of the Schrödinger equation and its expansion to include negative domains by using complex numbers makes it possible to posit the presence of 'confirmation waves' (CW) fitting the complex conjugate Schrödinger equation. While I may agree that a transaction is a genuinely stochastic event, I now disagree with the certainty that TIQM proposes that OW or CW do not obey a deterministic equation. Stochastic events are so complex in nature that they may give the human observer the appearance of being random in nature, until an instrumental measure is performed (double slit experiment). Experimental results based on completed transactions provide a reliable derivation of the Bohm Rule rather than assuming it exclusively applies according to the standard Copenhagen Interpretation (CI) of quantum mechanics (QM). However, the big challenge of proving if the transactional interpretation (TI) will ever be testable in the laboratory remains. I have other justifiable reasons to suspect that CI is incomplete by itself unless it incorporates transfinite cosmological as probable when the occurring events predicted are confirmed or have a biological survival value for the human species as briefly argued below. When both ontological and epistemological views are combined as an 'Epistemontological' unit it provides a more complete model, perhaps a theory of everything (TOE)? Why ignore events that history has recorded as 'belief' occurrences? They are existentially 'real' ontological facts regardless of their human interpretation as religions, cults, atheism, agnosticism, scientology, theosophy or what have you, a real conundrum!

My short quip answer to the conundrum is to recognize the superiority of sense phenomenal validation for ontological macro objects/events such as those we can experience if we walk inside the house blindfolded or, in a given moment we walk outside the house in a clear, starry night and observe the puzzling recursive cycles of predictable cosmological complex order we humans cannot control/influence and which cannot spontaneously be generated and sustained as also predicted by the entropy physical laws of nature. But just as convincing is the presence of those objects/events we all consistently, falsifiable and predictably experience that escape sensory detection or sometimes even a linguistic description? Are we justified in denying their vital presence in the existential reality of our environmental midst? Instead we can always explain their occurrence rationally using symbolic or sentential logic representations and using epistemological, mathematical logic tools, be they quantum logic and/ or conditional/Bayesian probability calculus. The arguments we have defended is that neither the physical phenomenological nor the metaphysical theoretical abstractions can exclude each other because they constitute a complementary/ functional unit whole to compensate for our human physical brain perceptual and conceptual deficits compared to other better adapted species sharing our biosphere environment.

While TIQM may not be currently testable in classical laboratories, that may be the consequence of our human technological limitations and should not be a deterrent to adopt because TIQM has been proven capable of generating new testable predictions on the basis of the probability of their occurrence as witnessed by the unrelenting march of technological and other complex developments. Keep in mind that even our most intelligent, better adapted chimp brothers and sisters can never accomplish that feat. In whose hands then are we leaving our civilization to develop as humans complete their life cycles? Do we have a responsibility for future generations? Or do we live just to satisfy the biopsychosocial (BPS) imperative that we share with other evolved species? The TI is not an exact interpretation of classical QM Bohm Rule and the Copenhagen Interpretation demands but, like the many-worlds interpretation (MWI), TI provides a logical physical map to follow with all the formal symbolic/sentential logic representations as a compass guide into a possible evolving reality as detailed in the Bohm Rule. It is a probable road map path to ideally explain that which the senses cannot describe as complexity continues its unrelenting evolutionary progression into the future.

Just as 'untestable' it appears now to be my proposed theoretical blueprint sub-model of a dark baryonic DNA/RNA receptor codon in neuron networks to bridge the connection between unidentified coordinates in transfinite n-1 dimension space-time and the human pre-motor neocortex attractor phase space. I hope it can be experimentally shown to control the reciprocal information transfer as detailed elsewhere and briefly mentioned here. This has been my incomplete partial reply to another challenge to the Copenhagen interpretation: "Where in space-time does a transaction occur?" So long as the brain dynamics map representation is not conceived as causally efficient in generating the neocortical tissue territory it is describing, as some radical theoretical exclusivists and religionists would have it to fuel hidden political agendas. IMHO, any justifiable explanation that works and can keep humans alive, biopsychosocially happy and socially accepted so (s)he can continue participating—to the extent of their inherited or acquired resources—across generations in the creation of this wondrous civilization that no other species can, is welcome.

Another causal efficiency issue has seriously challenged the consistency of the TIQM especially when combined with the super symmetry requirements of 'string theory' in its 'loop' variation mode. The formal arguments are beyond the scope of this brief presentation but a related explanation is available in the 'Twistor' theory. (See below) But first, we will briefly build the foundations of TIQM as modified and adapted to our own BPS Model of Brain Dynamics in the "Neurophilosophy of Consciousness." model-poem.

NON LOCALITY 'IDEAL' ARGUMENT

This is perhaps the most important and most controversial aspect of the TIQM model as it applies to the 'ideal' component of my own BPS model of brain dynamics. We need an explanation for the consistent, mysterious measurements correlations between the properties of distant systems that remain operationally linked through non-local influences across space and beyond human control where no light signal can travel. The best known example of the invisible micro link is provided by the famous Einstein-Podolsky-Rosen/Bohm (EPR/B) strongly suggesting it. In a nutshell, as seen in the diagram below, if subatomic particle spin pairs are separated and emitted in **opposite** directions from a source, they remain mysteriously entangled as measured by spin meters instruments capable of measuring spin components along various directions even when situated miles apart as shown below.

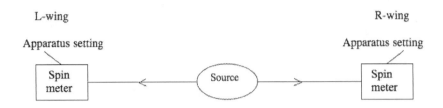

My own explanation, within the context of my proposed transactional reciprocal codon receptor in neurons linking/entangling/bridging a transfinite n-1 dimensional source and an acceptor brain site at the pre-motor neocortex. They are functionally coupled and influence each other by spin coupling as published in detail in "Neurophilosophy of Consciousness", Volume IV under "Speculations and Conjectures." Chapter I argues for the "Reciprocal Transactional Information Transfer Neocortex ←→ Transfinite" where neocortex refers to the 'real' local decision-making machinery in the premotor area of the human brain neocortex attractor phase space. Transfinite space refers to a set of 'ideal' n-1 dimensional transfinite non-local space set of virtual set of undefined spatial-temporal cosmological coordinates ***outside*** our local Minkowsky macro 4-dimensional sensory space. It all boils down to an (metaphysical) explanation and ***not*** an ontological (material physics) description of objects and events of experimental data measured in the Bell experiments when testing the Einstein-Podolsky-Rosen/Bohm (EPR/B) theory actually ***implying*** non-local events. The unexpected results suggested to me the possibility of a functional entanglement between the coordinates in the extrasensory cosmological non-local space-time realm and our local premotor area of the brain. The pre-motor neocortex contains subconscious memory stores of probable adaptive solutions to ongoing familiar problems which are considered before their conscious neuro-humoral mediated motor execution.

In my model the communication between a transmitter and a receiver is mediated via a receptor bridging a transfinity source of cosmic radiation and a brain premotor area receiver via a dark baryionic receptor transduction DNA/RNA codon. Cramer's original model explaining entanglement between source and destination was rudimentary and did not involve either the reciprocity feature or a mediator receptor of dark baryonic matter to mediate the local ←-→ non-local information transfer between coupled sources when Cramer studied the olfactory system. I modified Cramer's model by including reciprocal transmission and suggesting the dark baryonic codon mediator. This allowed me to extend the application beyond the olfactory system by generalizing the transfinite cosmic radiation effects to general modifications in the translation/transduction processing of genetic codons information into altered enzyme production without being detail-specific about any particular enzyme protein modification of its activity. The brain neuronal circuitry I proposed represented a cooperation between the local slow poke brain synaptic information transfer and the faster than light non-local source when synchronously entangled. This mechanism provided the means of spontaneous spin-spin coupling and synchronization we experimentally measure between transmitter and receiver are separated by great distances.

The details of the non-local effect suggests that the particles have a *random* spin when they leave the source in opposite directions and become linked in a definite spin orientation only with the first spin measurement implying that the outcome of this measurement is a matter of random chance. IMO a stochastic progression needs not to be random, only more difficult to ascertain its location experimentally. Be it as it may, if, e.g., the first measurement is set for a z-spin measurement on the L-particle, the L-particle will register a spin either clockwise (spin up) or anti-clockwise (spin down) about the z-axis (perpendicular to the 2-dimensional x-y plane) with an equal chance of producing an <u>instantaneous</u> change in the spin orientation of the distant R-particle by non-local spin coupling we call entanglement. The explanation is given as a 'collapse' of a traveling Schrodinger's wave function. In my view, the experimenter causes a collapse of a particle being carried by a wave (de Broglie's 'wavicle'), wherever that mass particle may be located. Particles generate waves or fields, waves or fields never generate particles in our human mesoscopic ontological experience, the only one that counts!

A proper human understanding of the TIQM model requires a special self directed introspective distinction between the "I" observer and that 'other' object/event being observed. This automatic effort allows you to adopt the proper perspective (framework of reference) before your analysis of any given object/event occurrence meanings. I feel there are too many brilliant people either paying too much attention to a branch of the tree and losing perspective of the forest or the reverse, generalizing too much about the forest ecosystem and not being very detailed about the specifics of a particular branch in a given tree. Or none of the above for the known listing trollers that joke or demonize with 'ad hominems' instead. :-) That distinction between 'I' and the 'other' will help to understand better what a 'wave function collapse' is. IMHO it was all about an attempt to explain the mystery of the Einstenian 'spooky actions at a distance' or non-locality requiring ultra luminal speeds. I call it a mystery because the Bell's speculations results from falsifiable, consistent probability-filtered measurements but lacking solid ontological/phenomenological underpinnings and thereby not amenable to experimental testing on its truth value certainty. But, sure as hell, perfectly valid to understand better spin-spin, matter-antimatter coupling and seemingly instantaneous phase synchronization between particles separated by distances measured in cosmological units. Here is the way I explain it to myself how the whole panoply of 'real' facts and fancy 'ideal' explanations about the TIQM model come together in a nutshell:

I will start with a reply to a well known theoretical mathematician/physicist from New Zealand who still challenges the necessary requirement of identifying at least the probable location of a causally efficient _**force**_ responsible for the consequent results he can only formulate in symbolic or sentential metaphysical, epistemological abstractions he swears by as an exclusive necessary and sufficient explanation, a radical view of exclusion. Here was my reply to a discussion of 'twistors' relation to the TIQM model theory when I challenged the necessary assumption of a *random* spin orientation of the particles when leaving the source in opposite directions of a stochastic/chaotic travel. (refer to figure above):

"Unless I am overlooking something important here, the causally efficient required force (f=ma) is accelerating a physical mass (m) spin particle being accelerated (a) when carried in a wave (de Broglie's 'wavicle') or across a magnetic field. Conservation of energy principles drives the particle (photon?) across the least resistance path as a spiraling 'twistor' to minimize the anticipated frictional resistance of a linear path. Light cannot exist without a source either the particle photon or an unidentified outside source (cosmic radiation from transfinite sources?). According to the twistor 'ideal' interpretation of the virtual reality theory (see diagram below) having the experimentally 'uncoupled' particle photon intersect at the cone vortex as they travel in opposite directions from the source analogous to (left ←→ right) linear travel away from the source as graphically shown before of the mass sub atomic particles wrongly assumed randomly uncoupled soon after leaving the source. IMO, what is important to notice here is that the accelerated mass sub particles *remain* entangled while they are carried by a wave or field whether electrical, magnetic or otherwise ('spooky' non-local action at a distance). Either way we choose to graphically represent the 'ideal' occurrence one of the sub-atomic particles is now in a negative domain after completing a full circular rotation in the 'twistor' model below or the 'linear' model above, as they sub-Planckian particles travel in opposite directions. This leads me to suspect that it instead complementary photon particles themselves the source of 'light radiation' through perhaps a nuclide radioactive(?) decomposition. Light needs a material particle to produce it, like other predicates of matter (shape, form, color, etc.)." Why does it need an initial measurement at either extreme of the probability spectrum location?

Why Epistemology. Finally, another argument about the necessary but insufficient exclusive consideration of the phenomenology-based Copenhagen Interpretation (CI) of human existential reality as opposed to the modified TIQM BPS model incorporating also the metaphysical aspects of our real time, ongoing human experience into a unit 'epistemontological' hybrid wholeness rooted on measurable human brain dynamics. This comes about because, as it seems, our lab researchers and arm chair theoreticians have neglected the obvious fact that ours is a human story of our lives narrated in our adopted language semantic structure, with all the implications of our human brain limitations in the cognitive epistemological explanations of those vital aspects of species survival we cannot describe adequately on a phenomenological/ ontological basis.

As it happens many times there are always many consistent invisible objects/ events in nature present that even escape linguistic explanations where no distinction is possible between the state of a natural object/event and what I cognitively know or could conceivably know about it because experientially there is only an awareness of its consistent and demonstrable presence by their causally-linked effects or qualia experienced. This is intrinsically the case for the distant n-1 dimensional cosmological macro object /events or the 4-dimensional micro objects/events about atoms and electrons, quarks and strings, we can only indirectly measure or consistently observe their effects that we then represent as metaphysical logic symbols to epistemologically substitute for the more reliable but absent phenomenology. Enter the TIQM model to reconcile the fundamentally conflicting positions of the phenomenal realism of the seen and the unquestionable presence of the unseen as developed in the unmodified Cramer transactional model poems and the necessary but incomplete physicalist positivism of the Copenhagen Interpretation.

Once we become aware of our human species comparative limitations in sensory and brain combinatory resolution of reality, it leaves open the question of whether or not there could be possible to have an absolute macro description of phenomenal reality as a fact. We can detail similar arguments to our conceptual explanations of physical reality below the threshold of human sensory resolution. We believe, however, that both analytical considerations can compensate each other's limitations and a hybrid Epistemontological theory is possible because the 'real' ontological descriptions and the 'ideal' epistemological explanations are incomplete when considered as exclusive of the other. As more technological information becomes available we need to dynamically integrate both aspects as we witness a transition from the 'ideal' to the 'real' circumstances of our human species limitations in cognitively analyzing the evolving complexity of our ongoing existence so we biologically survive across generations.

SUMMARY AND CONCLUSIONS

THE UNEXPECTED TRANSITION FROM IDEALISM TO REALISM

The information explosion we have witnessed in the last two decades has unexpectedly accelerated the relentless, forward evolutionary process of complexity as experienced and narrated by human language semantic accounts in our communications. There is an insurmountable amount of verifiable evidence sustaining the 'real' demonstrable fact that only the human brain and that of our <u>primate relatives</u> have the ability to pay attention to objects/events in the audio-visual scene without always looking or listening at them directly. This is done by recreating an internal map of the previous sense phenomenal world we experience by mapping our sensory field onto specific <u>brain cells</u>. The mapping includes local and non-local verifiable observables. This is the existentially **<u>real</u>**

case whether the 'wave' or 'field' mass particle carrier we conveniently derive as an **ideal** notion fits the previous consistent falsifiable experience or not. Thus, the local quantum physics interpretation implies being bounded within a finite space-time region where an observable object/event exhibits a 'real' behavior conditioned to the relevant environmental circumstances properly belonging to the space-time region itself. This is the classical Copenhagen Interpretation (CI). It is along these lines that the linear algebraic approach focuses on 'real' physical local and 'ideal' metaphysical non-local representations (symbolic or sentential logic) on a probability basis emphasizing that the notion of a field or wave is only a convenient derivative notion from the 'real' local actual measurements that preceded the 'ideal' non-local explanation.

The competing model-poems that 'ideally' explain the same 'real' phenomenological description of the object/event sensory reality that preceded it is called the Transactional Interpretation of Quantum Mechanics TIQM. The advantage of the transactional interpretation is, in my opinion, that it incorporates probable interpretations of ongoing verifiable existential experiences that are irreducible to linguistic coding in symbolic or sentential logic representations. It's emphasis on sense-phenomenal empirical 'reality' descriptions are more reliable especially when the Transactional Interpretation (TI) predictions are confirmed. Consequently the Lagrangian Quantum Field Theory (QFT) is our most empirically well-confirmed physical theory where the 'ideal' explanation of the metaphysical component of 'real' empirical object/events descriptions harmonize. The reliance on verifiable sensory facts excels in the expediency of calculations and their intuitive understanding because it is closer to phenomenological experimental manipulation in the physics lab. That makes the derived metaphysical 'ideal' model poem more credible when applying the theory to make predictions. Anytime that a pragmatic empirical 'reality' description of the occurrence of an object/event and an 'ideal' metaphysical logic sophistication explanation (i.e., there is an isomorphic mapping of the elements of a C^*-algebra into the set of bounded operators of the Dirac/Hilbert space.) lead to the **same** existential reality conclusion, then pragmatic 'realism' trumps mathematical rigor due to the resulting simplicity, efficiency, and ease in understanding. When the TIQM model is mathematically modified further to incorporate the speculative probability of identifying the n-1 dimension space coordinates of probable sources of cosmological information input located beyond our local 4-dimensional space-time, the TIQM becomes a superior 'ideal' model when also explaining non-local sources of information input (e.g., measurable cosmic radiation) causally efficient in influencing the human evolving complex 'reality'. This emphasis has made possible to grasp the seemingly conflicting multidisciplinary aspects of the same human reality in a real mesoscopic biosphere vital environment. This has been my personal experience.

The TIQM model superiority is best illustrated by adopting the Dirac <bra-ket> notation analytical tool, an empirically based 'ideal' representation where the 'entanglement' coupling is based on the complementary pairing/coupling of opposite spin unit particulate matter. The mechanism needs to be at the subatomic micro level but two macromolecules like DNA or RNA can be functionally coupled iff their micro components are spin-coupled first. I am not even sure that experimentally our sources are actually separating spin couples at random, it may be separating in opposite directions larger photon components already coupled that remain so even at cosmological dimensional units, as explained in the introduction above. We may never know. That way local or 'non-local transfinite information' input can gain empirical 'de facto' codon control of the transduction/translation genetic genotype machinery resulting in verifiable empirical phenotype results as observed in experimental labs as an induced re-arranging of the corresponding polynucleotide DNA helical structure and the subsequent RNA translation of environmental alterations in the corresponding functional enzyme production controlling phenotype expressions as briefly explained below in tracking the phenotype results from environmentally induced genotype alterations, e.g., 'optogenetic' tests.

It should be noted that the sophisticated mathematical axiomatic (logic) 'ideal' representation of the verifiable 'real' fact observation of an object/event in a derived wave or field conveyance regards the conveyance conceptualization as the fundamental notion for no convincing reason other than the symbolic/ sentential representational elegance. The 'ideal' elegant map sophistication has unjustifiably become thereby more important than the 'real' empirical observable territory! Thus, the Wightman axiomatic quantum field theory (QFT) becomes thereby superior to the linear algebraic QFT even when both are abstract explanations of an 'ideal' field with infinite degrees of freedom for putative sub-Planckian quantum particles that appear in special circumstances.

As noted earlier, the less mathematically elaborated algebraic QFT abstraction originated from observables in the measurable local and the probable non-local environments whereas the more mathematically sophisticated axiomatic approach is limited to a conceptual elaboration of the field, a derived carrier model notion from classical local quantum physics. Furthermore, in the classical local quantum physics interpretation an observable is regarded as a property belonging to space-time region itself, i.e., Higgs Bosons 'creating' something out of a nothing vacuum? Is this a new mathematical 'Genesis' criticizing the 'Delta Function' as improper and laden with self derived contradictions as Von Neumann opined?

Fortunately, as it turns out, von Neumann was the proponent of a new 'ideal' framework based on Hilbert's theory of operators and Dirac was the proponent of a 'real' framework of reference amenable to the rigors of testing of the local phenomenal events in the biophysical chemistry labs (e.g., optogenetic testing to cover the micro invisibilities) and the non-local events in the astronomy observatories covering the cosmological transfinite n-1 dimensional invisibilities.

Mathematically, the Dirac Delta Function is limited in scope when defined over the 'real' line, is zero everywhere except for one point at which it is infinite, and yields unity when integrated over the real line. Von Neumann promotes an alternative framework, which he characterizes as being "just as clear and unified, but without derived mathematical objections." He emphasizes that his framework is not merely a refinement of Dirac's; rather, it is a radically different framework that is based on Hilbert's theory of operators-valued distributions. When objectively, dispassionately analyzed both arguments have their own merits but would be incomplete if either one claims exclusivity. If we had to choose only one it is clear that when pragmatics and rigor lead to the **same** conclusion, then, as I said above, pragmatics trumps rigor due to the resulting simplicity, efficiency, and increase in understanding made possible. Most important, however, is that it allows for unexpected new environmental circumstances as they get empirically detected. In other words, the TIQM model approach adopts the pragmatic orientation in the Lagrangian QFT (based on perturbation theory, Feynman's path integrals and renormalization techniques). The "axiomatic" QFT refers specifically to the 'ideal' derived component of existential reality based on operator-valued mathematical distributions.

The undersigned author is not that familiar with the Weinberg 'real' pragmatic formulation that allegedly zeroes in human physical intuition and provides heuristics that are important when performing calculations; however, the mathematical theorists do not consider it mathematically rigorous enough and pay little attention to the fact that their proposed mathematical structure does not provide any techniques for connecting with familiar or new experimentally determined quantities. It is clear that these two approaches to QFT, the rigorous axiomatic and the Lagrangian pragmatic are rival research programs. I think we can get the best of both propositions that harmonizes with ongoing complex phenomenal reality as it evolves and I satisfy my curiosity as to their philosophical foundations. Then, because of my neurophilosophical interests in using the best available strategic tool when analyzing the mysterious struggle of our human species trans-generational survival against odds I compare the competing mathematical strategies and wonder why use the infinitesimals of classical quantum physics when you can use n-1 dimension transfinite parameters, more meaningful in the analysis of current existential reality.

Who, when leisurely meditating on the issues of life and human consciousness upon retirement, has not immediately reckon the relevance of particulate brain matter in reciprocal motion inside and outside a physical brain and the force(s) fueling the physical mass unit particles to exhibit dynamic reciprocal motion according to the well established laws of physics? It was all about analytically speculating how such **motion** carrying the invisible micro unit dimensional particle in a putative field (electric, magnetic or both) or wave conveyance can be explained best using the available mathematical logic metaphysics tools. Dirac's pragmatic approach proposed the equivalence of matrix mechanics and wave or field mechanics by using the Delta Function, an improvement on the original Hilbert Space use by incorporating scalar metrics definable in terms of the mathematical scalar's complex conjugate (a coupling/conjugation of a 'real' number + an 'ideal' imaginary number). That strike of genius makes possible to analogize such coupling with the still mysterious experimental non-local coupling of opposite spin particles (Φ is the topological anti-dual of Φ^x) at a distance when the source allegedly fired them in *opposite* space-time directions. The double slit experiments show their remaining entangled connectedness even when miles apart. As mentioned above, the stochastic nature of the physical particles as they travel in opposite directions until one of them 'randomly' selects one of various spin orientations available in the instrument after which the other particle mysteriously selects **only** the opposite complementary orientation, a 'spooky' action at a distance as relativity considers the result. I personally think they remained coupled when they left the source. Our human brain limits in both the perceptual and conceptual resolution capacities makes my speculation impossible to measure but neither is it justified to assume their original randomness. How else can we simultaneously measure the position of a unit mass particle 'm' being accelerated 'a' by a causally efficient force 'f' according to f=ma when the 'ideal' operators have no eigen values or eigen vectors? Here is the opportunity to calibrate the adequacy of competing mathematical physics 'ideal' algebras, one based on 'real' experimental observables related to bounded space-time locations like the finite double cone 'twistor' model where light traveling in opposite directions intersect at the vortex of the light cone or an 'ideal' algebra based on 'real' relativistic QFT interpretations? You be the judge, stay with the 'ideal' axiomatic version about how things should be (a la von Neumann) or transition to the 'reality' based version about how things probably are or predictably will be (a la Dirac), all things existentially relevant to human beings reality limitations being considered. Dirac's Hilbert space assigns generalized eigen functions to unit particle mass 'm' position and their instantaneous velocity 'v' from measurable F= mv momentum operators resulting in the nuclear spectral theorem where Φ and Φ^x remain connected as mathematically derived by an algebraic QFT of observables in our 'real' 4-dimensional Minkowski space-time.

Another instance for comparing the axiomatic or Dirac models is found in the recently reported "Breakthrough Study Reveals Biological Basis for Sensory Processing Disorders in Kids." As narrated, it constitutes the general explanation of the specific sensory processing disorders we clinically see in autism and the attention deficit hyperactivity disease (ADHD). It also underlines the importance of the human brain's right hemisphere first impact with sensory input from a 'real' phenomenological environmental (external or body proper) input sources of new or familiar information before an adaptive response is either subconsciously implemented reflexly or after further analytical processing especially when processing unfamiliar sensory inputs. It has been observed in the brain clinical lab how the **master** control nerve networks of the frontal brain neocortex is continually processing information input arising originally from the right ® hemisphere initial effort to coordinate ongoing 'real' phenomenological activity from multiple sources such as Left (L) temporal and parietal lobe convergence of multisensory input and Left (L) frontal language semantic processing Broca's area. The frontal neocortex brain is continually assessed of the whole spectrum of ongoing 'real' environmental biopsychosocial (BPS) relevant circumstances, from passive meditation to active social partying. When the new or familiar input is received at the Right hemisphere the master frontal neocortex analytical sorting of available response alternatives present in the neocortical pre motor attractor phase space working memory. This subconscious effort is subsequently followed by a conscious activation of the best adaptive motor choice neurohumoral response, all things considered. What is important to notice is how the brain synaptic 'real' time processing of information input precedes in time the freely conscious choice of the 'ideal' adaptive motor response. This choice is especially important in the presence of new/unfamiliar information sense-phenomenal input arrives in Right brain hemisphere. All of this complex analytical sorting immediately follows after a subconscious reflex motor response is released with priority for the overall biological preservation of the human species priority as previously published and discussed by me in various HiQ listings and fora. This detailed explanation hopefully supports my biased view about the importance of the 'real' preceding the 'ideal' solution. For more details see my Blog at: <http://angell.wordpress.com/>

When defending the human biological survival priority (BPS) premises as argued before the objections of some professional mathematical physics theorists, I state that by conditioning the sophistications of the axiomatic mathematical operations to conform the standard 'real' locality axioms e.g., isotony, locality, covariance, additivity, positive spectrum, etc., Dirac's original model theory can be extended to reach the cosmologic invisibilities of transfinite non-local space-time manifolds beyond our local Minkowsky 4-dimensional manifold. For the reasons stated above about the human species brain perceptual and conceptual resolution limitations, I am not including an unjustifiable inclusion of a mysterious and unique invariant vacuum state as already noted. This is the basis on which I am still working on an all encompassing TOE model poem of human mesoscopic existential reality incorporating and modifying the original Cramer's TIQM model and proposing the measurable details for the corroboration of a 'Transactional dark baryonic reciprocal receptor DNA/RNA mediating a two way information transfer between unidentified transfinite space-time coordinates and a premotor cortical acceptor in the human brain neocortical attractor phase space as published.

The resulting set of algebras on Minkowski space-time that satisfy these axioms is referred to as the *net of local algebras*. It has been shown that special subsets of the net of local algebras—those corresponding to various types of unbounded space-time regions such as tubes, monotones (a tube that extends infinitely in one direction only), and wedges—are type-III factors.

The classical N-dimensional complex vector space representation of a complete human brain dynamics of mesoscopic existential reality as the linear algebraic combination of the observable 'real' plus the logically inferred 'ideal' components waits for experimental corroboration of the putative 'reciprocal dark baryonic receptor' in human brain networks.

There is nothing new when we focus on our complex, evolving 'real' lives with the objects and events in our quotidian 4-dimensional Minkowsky space-time physical environment. A reliable simplification can be achieved if the 'ideal' component is dimensionally considered a vector $\mathbf{A}$ in an N dimensional vector space over the field of complex numbers $\mathbb{C}$, symbolically stated as $\mathbf{A} \in \mathbb{C}^N$. The vector $\mathbf{A}$ is still conventionally represented by a linear combination or sum (from n=1 to infinity N) of basis vectors as represented in a **column** matrix from A_1 to A_N:

$$\mathbf{A} = \sum_{n=1}^{N} A_n \mathbf{e}_n = \begin{pmatrix} A_1 \\ A_2 \\ \vdots \\ A_N \end{pmatrix}$$

even though the coordinates and vectors are all complex-valued by including putative negative dimensions to explain the 'transactions' between local and non-local cosmological coordinates.

We can improve on the reliability of such model if we avoid immeasurable infinities (N) and settle for probable transfinite n-1d approximations. This way, $\mathbf{A}$ can be a vector in a complex Hilbert space. Some Dirac/Hilbert spaces, like $\mathbb{C}^N$, have local **finite** dimension (d), while others have a non-local **infinite** dimension (n) adjustable to a **transfinite** (n-1 d) dimension so it becomes related to local sensory objects/events. In an infinite-dimensional space, the column-vector representation of $\mathbf{A}$ above would be a list of infinitely many complex numbers from A_1 to A_n as shown above. The symbol to the left, above, indicates that all n-dimensions are summed/integrated and may be represented as a **row** as seen below if represented as a $|B\rangle$ 'ket' B. Finite dimensions are experimentally testable for local observable/environmental 'real' conditions while transfinite coordinate locations are more adequate for probable testable non-local 'ideal' environmental situations especially for their predictable potential of future catastrophic events threatening the human species transgenerational biological survival against 'real' adaptive odds.

$$|A\rangle = A_x|e_x\rangle + A_y|e_y\rangle + A_z|e_z\rangle = \begin{pmatrix} A_x \\ A_y \\ A_z \end{pmatrix},$$

or in a more easily generalized notation,

$$|A\rangle = A_1|e_1\rangle + A_2|e_2\rangle + A_3|e_3\rangle = \begin{pmatrix} A_1 \\ A_2 \\ A_3 \end{pmatrix},$$

where the left 'bra' member is a 'row' and the right 'ket' member is a 'column' equivalent functionally linked. A bra next to a ket implies a linked/coupled matrix multiplication. (n x n). $\langle A| \times |B\rangle$

The bra row may be written in short as a ket row equivalent $|A\rangle = A_1|1\rangle + A_2|2\rangle + A_3|3\rangle$ or in any convenient symbol, letter or word inside the 'ket' column space. By common practice ket columns are used for labeling energy eigenkets in quantum mechanics with a list of their quantum numbers. In quantum mechanics, a **stationary state** is an eigenvector of the Hamiltonian, implying the probability density associated with the wavefunction is independent of time.[1] and thus the assumed invariant $\langle A|$ bra component in my 'ideal' 9-dimensional model of a 'complete' TOE model of human reality. The ket corresponds to a quantum state with a single definite energy (instead of a quantum superposition of different energies). The quantum states are _rays_ of vectors in the Dirac/Hilbert space, as $c|\psi\rangle$ corresponds to the same state for any nonzero complex number c. It is also called **energy eigenvector**, **energy eigenstate**, **energy eigenfunction**, or **energy eigenket**. It is very similar and equivalent to the concept of atomic orbital and molecular orbital in chemistry, with some slight differences as briefly explained below . . .

We use 'quantum numbers' to describe the micro spin values of conserved unit dimensional particulate matter quantities in the brain dynamics of the quantum system. Perhaps the most peculiar aspect of quantum mechanics is the quantization of observable quantities, since quantum numbers are discrete sets of integers or half-integers. This is distinguished from classical mechanics where the values are time-dependent variables and can range continuously. While quantum numbers often describe specifically the energies of electrons in atoms, they can also apply to angular momentum, spin, etc. as variables. Any quantum system can have one or more quantum numbers; it is thus difficult to list all possible quantum numbers.[1]

An inner product (n x n) is a generalization of the dot product. The inner product of two vectors is a complex number because it contains values in both the 'real' number positive and an 'ideal' virtual number negative vector directional domain. A bra-ket notation $\langle A| \times |B\rangle$ uses a specific notation for inner products. A bra next to a ket implies matrix multiplication. We can also use Dirac notation to represent inner or dot products.

One can also use the bra-ket notation to isolate different but related individualized sets of information content inside (brackets). $\langle A|B\rangle$ = the inner product of ket $|A\rangle$ with ket $|B\rangle$. If we analyze 'real' local verifiable environmental conditions inside our three-dimensional (3-d coordinate axes x, y, z at right angles from each other), a complex 9-dimensional Euclidean space is represented, the bra for a static, time-independent invariant situation and the ket portion representing the variable portion of the same reality represented in a linear metrics. The bra-ket representation takes the general form $\langle A|B\rangle = A_x^* B_x + A_y^* B_y + A_z^* B_z$ where A_i^* denotes the complex conjugate of A_i. We can easily see the 9-dimensional 'ideal' space come to life as published in more detail before.

Another important special case to notice is the inner product of a vector with itself, which is the square of its norm (magnitude) the bra-ket symbolic notation takes the row form $\langle A|A\rangle = |A_x|^2 + |A_y|^2 + |A_z|^2$

The real importance of the bra-ket notation is allowing the formation of **sets** confined inside (brackets) as when multiplying two sets of either stationary or variable quantities. $\langle A|B\rangle = (\langle A|)\,(|B\rangle)$. This way *both* the bra $\langle A|$ and the ket $|B\rangle$

are meaningful *on their own*, and can be used in other local or non-local contexts other than an inner or dot product representation. There is an obvious advantage about this ingenious way of representing the invariables and the variables, the local and the non-local, the 'real' and the 'ideal', the present as it verifiably **is** in the 'real' world and the probable future as it **may be** or the 'ideal' world should be as a goal, the immediate from the transcendental, the journey and the destination, the map and the territory. This clear distinction in the ongoing complex evolution of the human existential reality, confuses the lay and the experts, with subconscious or consciously deliberate results, but ultimately to protect human lives from eventual extinction after completing their life cycles.

Whatever the good, bad or indifferent intention to maintain our human biopsychosocial (BPS) integrity and keep track of the continuous relentless challenges in our environmental biosphere may be, we need an appropriate analytical logic tool allowing a continuous scrutiny of the present that is and the probable future that may or should be. The Dirac 'real' approach of focusing on the specific **physical**, verifiable observables using linear metrics represents to me the *necessary* frame of reference to **metaphysically** predict the probability of dangerous occurrences ultimately threatening human lives. The transactional interpretation of the quantum mechanics (TIQM) model, as modified, can accommodate relevant unsuspected occurrences. To follow is a brief account of the related sentential/symbolic linguistic representations in a linear algebra approach to vector calculus theory models.

The use of a scalar quantity metrics allows for the rigorous representation of intuitive geometrical notions such as the length of a vector or the angle between two vectors. They also provide the means of defining orthogonality between vectors of local environments, a scalar product of zero inner or dot product by generalizing our 3-d 'real' Euclidean spaces and also the probable 'ideal' vector spaces of any (possibly infinite) dimension, as are studied in functional analysis. Thus, there are finite-dimensional Dirac/Hilbert 'real' local spaces as fully elaborated in linear algebra, and there are n-infinite-dimensional separable 'ideal' non-local Dirac/Hilbert spaces that can be made structurally and functionally into n-1 dimensional isomorphic/equivalent to transfinite space $\ell^2(\aleph_0)$. Modified Hilbert spaces are Dirac space equivalents and there is a unique Dirac space up to isomorphism for every cardinality of the orthonormal basis. See below the vector notation for the xy plane

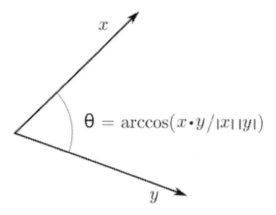

$$\theta = \arccos(x \cdot y / |x| \, |y|)$$

Dirac's bra-ket notation reliably makes possible a separation of the 'real' 4-d Minkowsky space-time describing what happens in the 'real' local dynamic human brain (as measured by fMRI and other techniques) from the 'ideal' non-local but probable and predictable n-1d _transfinite_ space conditioned to the elusive proof that every bounded linear operator on a Dirac/Hilbert space has a proper invariant subspace. In my biased opinion some cases of this invariant subspace problem have already been proposed along with my own published speculative arguments. A reconciliation of quantum and relativistic aspects of human existential reality has proven to be insurmountable, especially the mathematical conundrum of describing the sizes of infinite sets using the _transfinite_ cardinal numbers as briefly summarized now . . .

. The notion of using (brackets) is predicated on their ability to isolate as **'sets'** related aspects of one same human existential 'reality' some of which may be functionally linked (entangled) in the local or non-local environment. The cardinality concept was intuitively developed by Georg Cantor, also the originator of set theory, in 1874-1884. Cardinality can be used to compare two or more different finite sets such as e.g. the two sets {1,2,3} and {4,5,6} as having the same cardinality if combined and arranged to have a one-to-one correspondence reciprocal link between them {1->4, 2->5, 3->6}). When applied to **infinite** sets;[1] e.g. the set of natural numbers n = {0, 1, 2, 3, . . .}. now becoming denumerable (countably infinite) sets and this cardinal number is called $\aleph_0$, aleph-null also called transfinite cardinal numbers.

The magic of the TIQM Dirac's genius when handling the 'ideal' non-local environmental coordinates in n-1 dimensional transfinite space is to be able to 'see the unseen' objects/events by humans and make probable predictions and preparation strategies to protect against their potentially harmful future causal effects on human lives on earth. As mentioned above, the notation demonstrates how a bra can become an equivalent ket by way of a conjugate transpose (Hermitian conjugate) of a bra into the corresponding ket and vice-versa: $\langle A|^{\dagger} = |A\rangle$, $|A\rangle^{\dagger} = \langle A|$ because if one starts with the bra **row** representation: $(A_1^* \quad A_2^* \quad \cdots \quad A_N^*)$, and then perform a complex conjugation followed by a matrix transpose, one ends up with the equivalent ket **column** or vice verse as seen below:

$$\begin{pmatrix} A_1 \\ A_2 \\ \vdots \\ A_N \end{pmatrix}$$

Bras can become the linear operators on kets such as states whose <u>wavefunctions</u> are <u>Dirac delta functions</u> or infinite 2-d <u>plane waves</u>, pretty much like modified Hilbert spaces but more flexible in that it doesn't require normalization of wave functions in quantum states that assigns a strictly positive *length* or *size* to each <u>vector</u> in a <u>vector space</u>, a goal for the possible future. <u>Measurements</u> are associated with <u>linear operators</u> called <u>observables</u> on the Dirac/Hilbert space of quantum states.

The dynamic environmentally induced interactive variations in the unit-dimensional aggregates, like time independent static invariants of the unit dimensional physical particule are also be described by linear operators on the Dirac/Hilbert space. It should be noted that 'real' sense-phenomenal 'local' and describable information input is taken care of by the classic Hilbert space but verifiable 'non-local' objects/events beyond human threshold of resolution capabilities can still be 'ideally' explained as probable by the inner product which by definition is linear in the first argument and bounded as derived comes from the <u>Cauchy-Schwartz inequality</u>. The functional integration of the 'local' and 'non-local' elements provides a much more complete description of human existential reality as argued.

In the specific case of our speculative arguments on how the human brain dynamically analyzes and processes reciprocal information inputs from environmental local (including body proper) and non-local transfinite sources we conveniently normalize or scale the quantum wave function to = +1 when involving vectors or linear operators. We find how bra-ket notations best explains the causal link between verifiable observables and the predictable micro spin coupling, as amply discussed elsewhere. The local (albeit of an infinite scope) verifiable objects/events are discrete and countable (quantized). The non-local (infinite) are continuous and non countable but may become verifiable on a quantum probability basis.

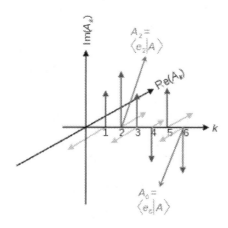

'Real' & local **discrete** with an infinite scope.

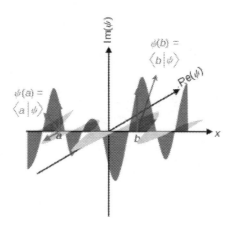

'Ideal' & non-local **continuous** with an infinite scope.

At the risk of being repetitious, we need to emphasize that any ket $|\Psi\rangle$ can *define* a complex scalar function of **r**, i.e., a wavefunction as $\Psi(\mathbf{r}) \overset{\mathrm{def}}{=} \langle\mathbf{r}|\Psi\rangle$ where $\Psi(\mathbf{r})$ on left is a mathematical function mapping any point in space acting on kets, by $A\Psi(\mathbf{r}) \overset{\mathrm{def}}{=} \langle\mathbf{r}|A|\Psi\rangle$, e.g., the momentum operator **p** in space **r** relates to wave function as $\mathbf{p}\Psi(\mathbf{r}) \overset{\text{def}}{=} \langle\mathbf{r}|\mathbf{p}|\Psi\rangle = -i\hbar\nabla\Psi(\mathbf{r})$. The Dirac/Hilbert notation may just as well explain the evolution of the complex brain dynamics when adjusting to ongoing familiar or new objects/events representing a potential threat to the human species biological survival as it causally affects its biopsychosocial (BPS) parameters.

One may conveniently consider a time independent unit dimensional discrete, invariant physical mass particle at a given moment in real time, mesoscopic existential reality as simultaneously coexisting with the corresponding time dependent continuous variations of their particulate characteristics as they aggregate in the same moment in time. The invariant infinite is countable by definition and the variant infinite is uncountable beyond the threshold of phenomenological resolution. They represent the entire spectrum of infinite reality from the micro sub-Planckian to the macro cosmological manifolds. Since infinite (N dimensional) objects/events are not phenomenological measurable in principle, we have to invent a putative countable transfinite (n-1 dimensional) manifold of discourse. The rest of the arguments will focus on the evolutionary component of the unit whole complex aggregate structure and function as anticipated and hopefully predicted and confirmed as causally related by their justifiable and consistent verification as probable. A transition from the unreliable indeterminate invisibility domain to the probable and more reliable determinate invisibility now able to be tracked in its evolutionary path with the mathematical logic tool of linear metrics that has proven so successful in science, technology and philosophy. We need to define the causally efficient force (f) behind acceleration (a) of the unit dimensional mass (m) particle responsible for their physical aggregates variations in structure and function (f=ma) affecting our existential human reality in our 9-dimensional biosphere environment as published elsewhere.

DIRAC'S VECTOR ANALYSIS UPDATE

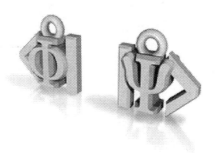

INTRODUCTION

Anyone who has ever stood up in front of a classroom to address his/her students will tell you that simplicity is a worthwhile pragmatic and theoretical virtue goal if and only the expected and appropriate pedagogic results are aimed at the student and not the teacher, independent of the corresponding level of complexity to be communicated. There is a presumption that 'selling/marketing' an idea by a professor implies there must be a 'buyer' student for a pedagogical transaction to be completed. Unless, of course, the professor, consciously knowing (or not) is engaged in a self-serving soliloquy justified as primitive, 'self-evident' propositions and often expressed as either theology or probable/statistical science inspired radical extremist pronouncements. Yet, a complex and changing nature, in its dynamic evolutionary progression in our 4-d space time existential reality, opts to reveal its complexity to human narrators in the form of the simplest possible model-poems solution that are compatible with the narrators' brain dynamics' phenomenology and combinatorial limitations, as amply detailed in our other publications. We now expand on the justifications for our general poem on the evolution of complexity as discussed under "The

Immanent Invariant and the Transcendental Transforming Horizons." See Ch. 12, "Nurophilosophy of Consciousness.", Vol. IV and Vol. V.

ARGUMENTATION

If we ever have expectations from our biopsychosocial (BPS) model poem of human brain dynamics ever evolving into a reliable theory of everything (TOE) it must satisfy some minimum requirements as detailed below. The most important requirement being that the model's principles must be rationally/ logically justified as a general/universal application to any aspect of human enquiry, whether its content is exclusively epistemological idealism or an exclusively pragmatic, methodological and empirical type. The model approach can also take the form of a hybrid combination of idealism and empiricism in nature like our own Epistemontological hybrid tracking this super-complex reality as it phenomenological evolves before our eyes in our 'real' 4-d space-time biosphere niche. We hope that our consciously free willed choice of simplified analytic mathematical elaboration is readable and reaches the curiosity of all informed readers in any discipline. In the search for an adequate universal mathematical formulation we had to justify the need for 'a priori' metaphysical elements (including philosophy, theosophy, mathematics, etc.) and the need for 'a posteriori' pragmatic/physical elements as emerging from scientific methodology measurements/observations of nature. It is due time to rationally integrate pragmatic 'real time' empiricism and rational idealism as a functional complete unit whole in living human mesoscopic reality as justified by consistent, falsifiable and predictable results from quantum theory based on probability theory and/or Bayesian conditional statistics calculus including theosophical-justified speculations and conjectures as exemplified by the famous Leibniz Monadology or our own sub-model arguments for the probability of a 'transactional reciprocal information transfer between the human pre-motor neo-cortex attractor phase space and unspecific space-time n-1 coordinates in transfinite as mediated by the human brain baryonic dark matter DNA/RNA receptor site.

Our central focus is on the human biopsychosocial (BPS) existential reality equilibrium adapting our species to familiar (or new) contingencies presenting a potential threat to the poorly adapted human biological survival. This puzzle has led us to seriously consider how may the human inferior adaptive limitations to a changing environmental landscape (compared to other evolved subhuman species) notwithstanding, the human species have survived across generations performing in the process the wondrous evolutionary technological and societal transformations other species are innately incapable of? What keeps the human species at the helm of the Bergsonian evolution of complexity; above and beyond the mere BPS survival that other evolved subhuman species also share?

Intuitively, the easy answer is to search for entities outside/beyond our immediate 4-d space-time earth biosphere environment that specifically/selectively influence the human species. The same intuition, always looking for simplicity, makes you posit the probability that before being the architect responsible for the wondrous transformation the human species has first to be alive, healthy and psychosocially adapted, in equilibrium with his immediate, individualized environment. It makes intuitive sense to suspect that such transfinite source should first be able to functionally equip humans with the resources to offset the inferior adaptive capabilities in the biosphere milieu and second 'create' the super symmetry transfinite conditions that minimizes the probability of disruptive transfinite radiation affecting our biosphere. Part of that radiation may exclusively reach the human pre-motor neo-cortex to anticipate the occurrence of damaging cosmic radiation events.

The careful reader may have noticed the posited existence of two unreachable infinities at play, the micro sub-Planckian manifold actively controlling the local events and the cosmological manifold controlling transfinite events. We immediately wonder what resources may our poorly adapted human species to life on earth, with its known phenomenal and brain combinatorial limitations, may mobilize to stay alive and become the architect of this wondrous civilization?? Can anyone imagine better adapted subhuman species like Rhesus monkeys or ants, roaches, etc creating optogenetic and gene transplant technology controlling DNA/RNA transduction, the same way transfinite radiation does? How else may any human being explain, if not describe, the cosmological order being influenced by natural complex asymmetries evolving to become the super symmetries that minimize universal damaging radiation impacting the earth and facilitating the reciprocal information transfer mechanism between humans and transfinite sources. We need a model poem formula that operates both at the local mesoscopic biosphere and at the cosmological order level that is compatible with the structural/functional idiosyncrasies of a human brain where our narratives become vital to continued survival against new or familiar negative odds . . .

We have climbed on the shoulders of Dirac and others to formulate probable approximations compatible with all disciplines created by the same human physical brain. What follows is a brief summary of the salient technical features still undergoing revisions with the joint 'help' of the good willed informed literati and the ill willed vicious strollers that plague some HiQ online listings. ☺.

For details on these formulations see Blog site: <http://angelldls.wordpress.com/>; and <http://delaSierra-Sheffer.net>. For the present needs of this brief article on the merits of a modified Dirac notation. We only highlight the possible interactive correlations between the local and transfinite sources of information and the need for functional approximations requiring a minimization of relevant interacting variables at both extremes of the spectrum, the phenomenological invisible levels of activity at both the sub-Planckian local level and the cosmological level. At the micro level our sub model requires the attainment of super symmetry to posit the presence of monopoles and gravitons to facilitate the influence of low intensity transfinite cosmic radiation on the local genetic transduction process of the brain neuron target cell via a dark matter baryon receptor. The ongoing debate centers on what subatomic micro particle is involved in the information transfer, the neutrino, the axion, etc. and where does it originate? We concentrate on the measurable how and give a lower priority to the theosophical why.

The charge free 'neutrino' is the candidate of choice to penetrate un-opposed miles deep through geological barriers to reach the buried instrument receptors at CERN. Radioactive, stable hydrogen H_1 (spin 1) atoms are known to spontaneously emit ½ spin electrons during their Beta decay process to a suitable acceptor of opposite-1/2 spin configuration leaving the originally stable spin 1 source spin—½ deficient as allegedly measured. In our model this naturally decaying or cosmic radiation-induced hydrogen atom can be on either side of the reciprocal communication path spectrum, the human brain cell or a transfinite source of radiation. It is assumed that path direction is a function of need to insure the availability of an BPS survival adaptive response to challenging environmental contingencies. All experiments confirm the same fractional deficit attending radioactive degradation. If, as the result of nucleosynthetic activity immediately after the Big Bang, dark baryonic particle radiation found its way into cellular DNA/RNA is not as farfetched as it seems to arm chair idealist theorists who rather prefer the charming argument of the 'mass less' physical particle <http://en.wikipedia.org/wiki/Weyl_equation> to justify the deep penetration of the particulate matter. Somehow the 'mass less' particle has to be charge-neutral and only micro gravitational forces in the form of magnetic monopoles will do to avoid the dipolar nature of electromagnetic (EM) induced fields. Can a counter intuitive 'mass less' particulate matter induce EM fields?

Enter gravitons and Dirac who questioned what good theoretical reason explains why the un-observed/undetected monopoles could not exist within a quantum theory framework? A mathematical logic explanation made more overall sense to posit the existence of monopoles than its absence. It is clear that a consistent, falsifiable observation or a physics-laboratory experiment should not necessarily be always considered as a check on the necessary and sufficient proof of its truth content. In our opinion the same incompleteness applies to the conceptual mathematical correctness of the symbolic or sentential representations of the current Dirac-equation solution. However, when both the physical empirical measurement of a consistent/falsifiable effect and a metaphysical logic are integrated, the confirmation of the electron particle physical mass, graviton or monopoles structure become a goal whose detection ability in the electron physics lab is still beyond reach, if ever, but at least its predictions on a probability basis is the next best option.

The best way to explain the temporal evolution of the multidimensional complexity of any quantum state in a linear scalar progression (the same way our brain linearizes sensory information input) is to update the Schrodinger and Hamiltonian space into a Hilbert space that may take into account any vector ray projection path direction. This mathematical combination allows for the differential representation of a multiple number of relevant variable paths interacting between themselves as one single resultant package. Each of the participating quantum states can be represented in the standard 'Bracket' notation $\langle \phi | \psi \rangle$. $\langle \phi |$ is called the bra and a right part is called the ket $| \psi \rangle$. The <bra-ket> notation was invented by Paul Dirac. The effective use requires minimizing the number of relevant dependent variants by approximations as they affect the phenomenological perceptualization of an independent invariant unit dimensional physical particle or aggregations thereof. In a TOE model any conserved value, matter, momentum, etc. will do as the invariant. It should be remembered that the progression range of all of the N particles (positive integer; 0) individual 3-d x, y, z dependent variables inputs as they project into a Hilbert space of 6N real dimensions gets reduced to a single valued function output. Quantum theory integrates the 3-d configuration space plus the 6-d Hilbert space into a 9-d space may now 'represent' the classical brain phase space. This way each projective ray path projection represents a frame-independent Schrodinger wave function where the operator defines the appropriate frame of reference. If one path harmonic ray rotates, stretches, etc., they all do (at right angles to each other or orthogonal) except when several points cohabit and interact in same 2-d plane (not the x, y, z line axis!) where each point coordinates lies (each Eigen value, momentum, position, spin, etc. defining its probability amplitude) may have conflicting physical existence. Not all possible observables can be simultaneously measured, eg., position and spin of particle, giving rise to Heisenberg' uncertainty principle. At the sub-Planckian scale (10^{-33} cm) quantum gravity space is a lattice and we can have an infinity of dimensions for an open ended forever-expanding universe. Each of these mutually perpendicular basic rays represents a particular potential behavior of a quantum system and the set of all basic rays for a given property constitute the relativistic frame of reference in Hilbert space. Orthogonal spaces provide for potential activities that are classically distinct or mutually exclusive. Also, the number of dimensions needed in this abstract space corresponds to the number of choices available for the quantum system, and this, as we have just seen, can go to infinity. In such cases the product of their Hilbert spaces gives rise to the "entangled states" of the Einstein-Podolsky-Rosen/Bohm (EPR/B) effect. In Hilbert space the ubiquitous electron can be in all possible places all the time. In this respect a Hilbert space concept is more than adequate to carry on the baton for the representation of the quotidian familiar everyday world.

In general terms the Dirac notation satisfies the identities inside the brackets as detailed at http://en.wikipedia.org/wiki/Complex_conjugate_representation outside the scope of this brief presentation. By mathematical logic transformations the general terms can be further transformed into operational functional representations allowing a 'visualization' of the temporal course of evolution of any unit dimensional invariant particle aggregates as they project their evolutionary progression into the multidimensional Hilbert space allowing for predictable warnings about probable future happenings in our biosphere of interest.

SUMMARY AND CONCLUSIONS

If the objective reader still considers recorded history as at least a reliable guide as to how complexity has evolved from memorable Aristotelian times to our convulsive 21th. Century, it should be obvious that each historical period had the task to reconcile the immanent/pragmatic, phenomenological 'seen' and the transcendental, relevant epistemological 'unseen'. We can summarily mention Aristotle's analytical guide in his 'ceteris paribus' strategy to minimize the number of postulates or hypotheses to make your model poem more credible. Even St. Thomas Aquinas recognized in the Middle Ages how natural laws of simplicity adequately guide the course of universal evolution. Likewise Kant—in the Critique of Pure Reason—supports the idea of minimizing the number of non-phenomenological assumptions/principles contained in 'Pure Reason'-based arguments underlying scientists' theorizing about nature. If true and sufficient, as consistently verified by all human observers, whether philosophers, experimentalists, and/or practitioners, why muddle the truth content goal with the claim of exclusivity based on pronouncements about subjective radical sensory or extrasensory individualized experiences? Why not heed today the pragmatic, universal suggestions from 14th. Century's Occam's razor, Galileo or Newton's Principia Mathematica? Why settle for the self serving pomp and circumstance of superfluous causalities as defended by the radicalized arm chair physicalist theorists or the experimentalists, practitioners and philosophers? On the other radical extreme, why should anyone accept as the exclusive truth the metaphysical, subjective, individualized content of a physical human brain's theosophy-inspired cosmogony experiences? Three centuries ago the chemist Lavoisier ridiculed the hypothetical metaphysical 'phlogiston' as the exclusive explanation of phenomenological chemical reactions observed, a rejection based exclusively on mathematical logic principles that minimizes the arbitrariness of non phenomenal brainstorms. Again, mesoscopic existential reality demands the easiest and simplest explanations to explain the realities a healthy physical human brain experiences. To guaranty the maximum probability of truth content we need to integrate the maximum number of empirical consistent, falsifiable human measurements/observations resting on logical deductions and a bare minimum of axiomatic-based model poems. This is true of all disciplines created and narrated by the exclusive, individualized human brain dynamic activity whether we like it or not. The polarization we witness between the hands-on physical ontologisms and the armchair metaphysical epistemologists in current 21st. century debate on 'consciousness' seem to rely exclusively on the burden of proof summoned in defense of one's point of view, thanks to the magic experimental results coming from modern technology, especially when they score high in the predictive value. All things being hopefully considered, the undersigned author still believes that providing credible arguments rooted on solid consistent measured/observed empirical facts refuting competing theories is more important as a starting point in the debate as to the probable truth content of our conscious model choice. A case in point is the un-necessary causality debate on probable truth content between the undeniable linguistic elegance of armchair mathematics theorists and the hands-on cold probable/ statistical laboratory facts reports of real time-space practitioners. Considering the evolving super complexity of both the physical human brain structure/ function and that of the universe how dare either extreme version proclaim the exclusivity of their domain of discourse at the exclusion of the rival unknown other? Why do materialist physicists knowingly posit the existence of two coexisting but different ontologism in the mind-brain dualist interpretation of the human brain dynamics when they should know that etymologically ontology belongs to the phenomenological domain whereas mind is an epistemological denotation? Why not share and learn from each other including the justifiable arguments of each other in a current but evolving hybrid Epistemontological synthesis as we have proposed and have exhaustingly analyzed in our BPS model of brain dynamics.

The reason we briefly discussed the Dirac methodology is because we also believe that if our model aspirations of becoming an universal theory of everything (TOE) we should justify the BPS model poem of brain dynamics as applicable to any area of human enquiry regardless of being formulated as an epistemology or methodology principle because we consider both principles as two coexisting, inseparable aspects of the same mesoscopic existential reality in our human species biosphere.

Finally, I will try to dissect out for the more sophisticated reader the linguistic distinction between 'pure' and 'practical' as opposed to 'pure reason' and 'practical reason'.

The English semantic structure of the **noun** 'pure' implies an abstraction. When used as an **adjective** it modifies the noun, as in 'pure reason' where the focus is in the **noun** 'reason'. A careful reading of Kant will make it obvious that he never doubted that the activity of reasoning took place in a living physical brain. Mind and brain were used interchangeably as if the terms were indistinguishable from each other. Remember that the histophysiology (structure/function) of the brain was in its infancy in the 18th. Century before Nobel Prize winner Ramon y Cajal's nominal work on the brain's cyto-architecture. Ergo, Kant was focused on the epistemological activity of reasoning taking place in a physical brain. What did Kant say about reasoning?

What made Kant famous in philosophy was his famous "Critique of Pure Reason" where he convincingly argued that it makes no sense to reason about 'pure abstractions' beyond sensory resolution, like winged angels, spirits or their equivalents. He stressed that it was more credible and reliable to reason and describe sense-phenomenal physical objects and/or events others could corroborate. This is the empirical, ontological and pragmatic approach. What did he say on reasoning about the physical presence of falsifiable, reproducible and consistent object/events, such as a strong, wet, hot wind from the southeast across the lake causing my roof tiles to blow away and my porch door to break (a real case a month ago!)?. This what he said:

Absent an ontological observable account of a **describable** causally efficient agent, the brain (or mind) can always reason or **explain** the physical presence of a possible entity causing the described ontological results. The explanation accounts for the recorded elements registered, directional coordinates, temperature, humidity, wind speed, etc. All of this data is available to the brain to evaluate and predict future similar events based on memory recalls of similar occurrences when present. This brain mapping representation is made possible because we have a language capable of translating the observables into symbolic or sentential logic or intuitive equivalents. This abstraction becomes the epistemological model, the result of the brain's reasoning activity. The resulting abstract model is subject to confirmation or rejection as the environmental contingencies evolve. Please notice how ontological phenomenology precedes epistemological explanations according to Kant. Some may ask, then why did Kant write another "Critique on Practical Reason" years later? Did he change his mind? What did a more mature Kant have to say about practical reason?

He was actually talking now about the ethics and morality of relying exclusively on empirical, practical aspects by humans when their perceptual and conceptual brain processing limitations are taken into consideration as compared to other species. He was suggesting that, all things human being considered, including his evolving complexity, emotional, rational, etc. vis a vis the evolving complexity of his vital space environmental circumstances (communities, migrations, weather, etc.) it would behoove human survival potential the possibility that making decisions based exclusively on practical reasoning may be wrong if all relevant facts were known, such as mental capacity, health, or deliberate conscious lying by a narrator. He was suggesting that, as we are drummed in law school, it is better to let the guilty go free than deprive an innocent of his liberty, family, etc. Kant was accentuating the real worth of living with ethical and moral standards.

Kant did not have the advantage of modern technology, in vitro and in vivo, and couldn't appreciate many relevant issues like existential reality in a mesoscopic world. That is where we take over in our Epistemontological hybrid model of brain dynamics.

To exemplify how this transition from the 'ideal' to the 'real' BPS reality read the novel that follows after the References.

REFERENCES

Maudlin (1996, 2002) has demonstrated that TI is inconsistent.

Berkovitz, J. (2002). ``On Causal Loops in the Quantum Realm," in T. Placek and J. Butterfield (Ed.), Proceedings of the NATO Advanced Research Workshop on Modality, Probability and Bell's Theorems, Kluwer, 233-255.

Cramer J. G. (2005). "The Quantum Handshake: A Review of the Transactional Interpretation of Quantum Mechanics," presented at "Time-Symmetry in Quantum Mechanics" Conference, Sydney, Australia, July 23, 2005. Available at: http://faculty.washington.edu/jcramer/PowerPoint/Sydney_20050723_a.ppt

Kastner, R. E. (2006). "Cramer's Transactional Interpretation and Causal Loop Problems," Synthese 150, 1-14.

Marchildon, L. (2006). "Causal Loops and Collapse in the Transactional Interpretation of Quantum Mechanics," Physics Essays 19, 422.

Daniel F. Styer, Miranda S. Balkin, Kathryn M. Becker, Matthew R. Burns, Christopher E. Dudley, Scott T. Forth, Jeremy S. Gaumer, Mark A. Kramer, David C. Oertel, Leonard H. Park, Marie T. Rinkoski, Clait T. Smith and Timothy D. Wotherspoon (2002) "Nine formulations of quantum mechanics," American Journal of Physics 70, 288-297.

Family Domain site: <http://delaSierra-Sheffer.net>

Blog site: http://angelldls.wordpress.com/; <http://angelldls.wordpress.com/author/angelldls/> Books published: <http://bookstore.trafford.com/AdvancedSearch/Default.aspSearchTerm=neurophilosophy>; <http://www.facebook.com/pages/Dr-Angell-O-de-la-Sierra-Esq/187843051348771><http://www.lulu.com/shop/search.ep?keyWords=Dr.+Angell+O.+de+la+Sierra&categoryId=100501>

"Remembering John Arthur"

A virtual chronicle of a consciously willed suicide defying all laws of nature that guarantee the unavoidtable biological survival imperative.

The "I did it my way" strategy as the ultimate expression of a consciously chosen freedom. What forces motivate/drive a healthy freely conscious, good willed, loving, good looking young man to sacrifice his life for no known emotional or rational reason? How can anyone defy natural laws and the unconscious, genetic, powerful drive to comply with the biological imperative to survive at all costs?

CHAPTER

1

Dear Daniel, Barbie, Nini, my surviving brothers and sisters, Angell Jr. wherever you may be in a better world in heaven than that grayish looking prison room at Sullivan St. that Suzi re-Mom chose for us after marrying Daddy. I am sure none of you—or me included—will ever understand why, I had my named brand fashion style, the latest computer soft and hardware gadgets, smiled and happily strummed my electric guitar while at the same time consistently refusing medical help for my platelets production dysfunction which eventually I knew will cause my death from internal bleeding, like Daddy kept repeating and repeating to me in frustration, like a daily litany. He doesn't seem to understand that I want to be independent and self sufficient like he is and wanted all of us to be. If it is true that every time you depend on someone else you surrender that precious freedom in proportion to your degree of dependence. Why does he not get it?

What you are about to read below is a rambling rationalization of living experiences I never try to interpret or understand myself. Like a feeling of impending doom I could not stop or change its evolving path into an uncertain future with no lights to be seen at the end of the tunnel. So why not have fun doing things 'my way', look up at the Central Florida skies and hopelessly wait for miracles that I knew beforehand that will never happen.

Just bear with me, I will be bragging a little, sometimes crying a lot after several green Heineken beers, as I continue to live and let live while I wait with a smile for the inevitable course of events with contrived happiness and a smile, I wanted to do it my way. But please promise me you won't read this account of my controversial life until I am buried or cremated as the case may be. Who cares anyway, life continues.

There is not really an awful lot you don't already know about the circumstances surrounding my lifetime travels with Mom and Dad before you were even born and afterwards, but there are a few details that really made a difference, especially those living like a spoiled brat inside the State University of Puerto Rico campus premises inside Henry Barracks military camp in Cayey, Puerto Rico, which you are yet unacquainted with. And, of course, how they evolved after that frustrating, yet delightful experience with my girl friend Alejandra. The rest that followed in New York City, Long Island, New York, Spain, and Maryland happened before Nini was born. But none like the experience In Macondo, USA when I was exposed to the Spanish language for the first time during my pre-teen years. They have forever shaped my character by providing ethical and moral standards from various available perspectives to choose from as my guiding torch into the uncertainties of an always uncertain future. Do you remember when Alejandra, my Chilean next door girl friend in Henry Barracks . . . .

No, it is not either about little made-up anecdotes of Alejandra's ancestors, who the hell cares about who or where they originated from, Italy, Argentina's pampas or what have you. Really, who cares, as Daddy said? Neither is it about the relative intellectual elite and social prowess into which her family claims they were born and bred when growing up in the mountain slopes. Or their dislike for the Argentineans, their natural enemies north of Chile's national boundaries where Santa Pinter, our other Argentinean-Hungarian neighbor comes from. They all came as an intellectual elite feeling superior to the local jibaro professors. That sheltered, comfortable life we all enjoyed inside the campus contrasted with the other life outside the sheltered bubble routine playing with my poisonous spiders across the house and day dreaming about my Alejandra and the future together. Life outside campus with my broken Spanish and my implied special status as son of an Irish 'gringa' and the Dean of Natural Sciences was confusing in a town where mixed feelings existed about the drunken gringo soldier's invasion of town when headquartered at Henry Barracks Camp where we now lived. Following our parent's tradition of humility I mixed easily with everyone. I still remember all the English family names the gringo soldiers' rampage in town were responsible for, like Sullivan (now Solivan), O'Neill, etc. I didn't get a chance to reflect much on this conflicting psychology still co-existing outside campus until our whole family moved like a unit back to continental U.S.A. Our father had always said we wanted us to settle down and grow under the influence of a much older Spanish Catholic culture compared to continental U.S.A's mere 250 + years of constitutional and cultural unity experience. I always thought we'd follow the example of our campus neighbors who still today live in the suburban areas there. I thought we would settle down to live either way up near the central range of mountains at retiring Prof. Pio Lopez farm sharing a simultaneous view of the Northern Atlantic Ocean and the southern Caribbean Sea. Or else the farm Daddy purchased from his family vast control of flowering land sloping down the sides of El Yunque natural reserve. If you remember it was all covered with flowers carefully cultivated for sale. Instead, we ended up in Deltona, Central Florida where we still live near Lake Louise. That eventual transition upon Daddy's retirement from Academia to a more leisurely lake-front retirement comfort trying to share with other academics in cyberspace what would become his obsessive compulsive drive to explain life and consciousness had changed life for me in a dramatic way. I was supposed to enjoy living and sharing my sheltered conservative upbringing with others, perhaps way up in Barrazas, Carolina or at Pio Lopez farm. What happened? Daddy had grown frustrated with both the politicians-for-sale characters of the long-chained colony and the continuous, never ending flow of illegals from everywhere in the western hemisphere, even from China, all living without paying a penny in taxes he said. Mom also wanted to return to the mainland even though she successfully completed a degree in law at the best state university, in Spanish no less! She thought she would always care for us and, like Daddy, she thought that what God had especially given to you is not meant for self-indulgence but to improve the world you found according to your guiding religious faith and your faculties, those innate or acquired. Could I follow and succeed walking inside those same shoes and firmly take the same footsteps eventually? I don't know that was meant for me, I wanted to marry Alejandra and settle down on top of those beautiful mountains. This was not much to offer others but if I am not taking it from others, why not, like Daddy said. But, above all, I wanted to do things my way. I don't know if my relative successes in the real world are worth sharing with others, like Mommy always said, "your daddy's life plan is a tough act to follow". After dear Mom's untimely death shock. that I will never recover from, I know, what else is there for me? And honestly, if given an opportunity to reincarnate after my upcoming death, I would still reenact the same life style and do it my way.

Now and then, still unemployed, I tried to find my peace by hours spent strumming my electronic guitar trying to compose something original while Chevy Boy meows trying to climb on my lap. I relax a little and think again about Alejandra, the mountain top, you and our parents, then, looking back in time, I realized I had done pretty well by myself as a human being. I never expected any reward I hadn't earned by hard work and careful consideration about somebody else being hurt in the process. That lesson we all learned early on from our parents has guided my steps throughout my entire life. I can still see Daddy still scrutinizing my facial expressions and body language trying to read the words I am not verbalizing about my negative attitude towards being helped with my bone marrow problems. He must have been crazy to think he could have changed my mind because the die was cast. I could watch him crying in silence in desperation and I compassionately feigned compliance with my medication's schedule. He was put in my life for me to learn and follow his steps after he died and now I am dying first before his eyes and he doesn't know what to do about it. There were not enough platelet transfusions or expensive liver transplants to reverse the inevitable God's design. After donating a kidney to Angell, Jr., now barely surviving dialysis with terminal kidney disease, he felt helpless. But, in my mind, the die was irreversibly cast. I am sure he never expected to bury me first during the next weeks or so, to be followed by Angell, Jr. soon afterwards, considering the way things are going with him now, intravenous ports, infusions, transfusions, you name it! It was heart breaking to watch his tears cascading down his cheeks away from us to watch but other than feign compliance there was nothing else I could do either. In retrospect, I have been so lucky and blessed that I wouldn't have significantly changed much of my behavior to others or correct any major judgments on my sibling brothers and sisters other than natural sibling rivalries of planned short duration or my attitudes towards the needy, children, neighbors or pets, especially the latter. For life is all about love and needs first and not un-affordable conveniences, in that order. Stoic, sad, antisocial, shy introvert, ultrasensitive, witty, moderate, down to earth, a veritable carbon copy of daddy's mold . . . , yes all of those things, some loved, hated or felt sorry about by others, but I never had enemies. The only thing I have missed is not being able to marry Alejandra, lived up in the mountains with her and our children, continue to work in the hotel administration business or caring for pets in some animal hospital and then head home, play the base guitar, the piano or pet my animals to death. Like Daddy and Mommy, I got along better with animals than with people, especially the macho male wannabees in their never ending monologues about their sexual activity, leisure trips or business earnings. Like Daddy always said about our family, we are all living mostly inside protected sheltered lives inside spherical bubbles and we need to incorporate what the information explosion technology—that I was so familiar with first hand—has added to our decision making process. But it was getting too late for me, I am dying slowly and may not be even able to finish these farewell notes to you, my dear survivors to be. Needless to say that sometimes I wished I could stay to continue to experience the wondrous delight of our household zoo of dogs, cats, cranes, egrets, blue jays and buzzards, as I watch in awe both from the porch inside and the lake flora outside. I guess I will have no choice but to remain inside the spherical bubble and miss the new dimension of wisdom our father claims to have learned when he widowed and remarried our 're-mom' Suzi, the beautiful, fashion model and Baptist Deaconess who spontaneously provided that motherly shoulder for Daddy to incline his head on and dried his cascading tears when our brother died weeks ago now.

CHAPTER

I don't know if by now you all feel bored with these little details about me, probably Angell Jr. is yawning. Angell Jr. and I were always together until that unexpected special day when he announced that he was not going to attend college where an honor registration was waiting for him because of his high score in the entrance examination. He did even better in the Aswap military aptitude test. He didn't tell anyone in Cayey, including our family, that he was headed to an elite electronic training school in Chicago, not far from where the Irish end of Mommy's family still lives and Mommy grew up and graduated from St. Catherine Catholic College. Angell Jr. had mentioned to me about the electronic school but I was sure he would follow along by going to the state university all of us did and enjoy the financial benefits and considerations that usually come along for the children of faculty members. But his mind was made up. He loved electronics ever since he curiously watched Daddy tinkering and fixing equipment he had designed and put together himself in his lab. Angell Jr. loved assembling and disassembling all kinds of ships, airplanes, and other wooden models, as you know. What I never told any of you was that, during that memorable farewell trip we all made from Henry Barrack campus in our SUV to the San Juan International Airport to have Angell Jr. take a plane to his Navy temporary duty station assignment in Chicago, I had the distinct feeling that was the beginning of a trend that materialized when we all went back to continental USA in Deltona, Central Florida. Good bye Alejandra, good bye tall mountain side, good bye to the Caribbean Pearl of Puerto Rico . . . . good bye life . . . . Daddy said I didn't have to go with the rest of the family because I had a job, relatives living there and beauty all around those central range of tall mountains. But I knew he was lying as his eyes became again watery and he turn his head to avoid been seen. I will forever remember that trip where my father sobbed in faint but audible sounds as he drove to the airport and back to Cayey. Remember? Everything changed for me from then on. The die was cast and I decided to survive, however transiently, by doing things my way.

So many times thereafter I was surprised to find myself in front of a mirror in the solitude of our house bathroom subconsciously acting out a soliloquy of sorts inspired mostly by a contrasting and confusing combination of teary sorrow and vanity stemming from my music theory success in transposing music from the piano to the base guitar, a sort of balancing/neutralizing, ephemeral and self-serving indulgence? Such are the combinations of pleasures and sadness. A strange feeling of a vanishing dream, the prelude of an obligatory transmigration to the unknown took control of my mind. Interestingly, that is the same odd combination of pleasure and pain that often resulted in creative works of art in music, paintings, literature, etc. But I felt I did not have what it takes to succeed. It was the sort of creative vanity that leads you to challenge and control the impossible and the invisible like our crazy father. But I was more like our mother, quietly earning everybody's love by being soft spoken, maybe not so intelligent but quiet and compassionate like she was. I was not inclined nor empowered with the push genes to read, read and read until you are enabled to wrestle complexity down to symbolic or sentential logical representations you then hope to communicate intelligibly to reveal their inner structural/functional secrets. Life, after all, may just be an illusion and illusions are just that . . . , illusions. Perhaps I was caught in the middle of a vortex created by the many worthy and inconclusive projects my upbringing family experienced and now wished me to complete . . . . but I cannot because I wanna do things my way. I cannot lead or even participate, like, for instance, the Bobonis transplants from the Mediterranean Corsica, on Daddy's side, that played such an important role in the founding of Carolina, at that time just a palm tree haven in mid northern coastal Puerto Rico. Neither could I have migrate from County Mayo in Ireland to settle and successfully bring up a stable, loving, law abiding family in St. Paul, Minnesota as exemplified by our mother. It is not my cup of cake, I am a peaceful, scared follower, the reason I followed the rest of the family back to continental USA leaving behind my dreams and hopes in beautiful Puerto Rico . . . sorry about that, C'est la vie, C'est la guerre . . . . It is funny how members of the same ethnic tribe, so to speak, with same habits, religion, biases and even natural intelligence potential pursue different paths in their lives, some come to give and share, other to receive and keep. How are they selected?. We see that in both sides of our family. The one's giving and sharing are more reserved, shy and quiet introverts whereas the one's receiving and keeping are usually outspoken extroverts paying more attention to external appearances and success. From Daddy's side, you know about the many such Corsicans, now mostly headquartered in the southwestern tip of the island who could have actively participated in the early Carolina settlement & development but they didn't. Instead they rather conveniently chose to claim a special status because of their ethnic Sub-European/Mediterranean origins, where Napoleon was born! These are the tribal things that can only flourish in modern colonial Macondos where Arawak Indian aborigines and African slave descendants are still looked down upon. On the other end of the spectrum are the other Bobonis family members who became lawyers, professors, physicians and dentists we were all so proud of or even other self educated achievers like Daddy's uncle Agustin, who with only a high school diploma and an insatiable lust for books and knowledge no one could match, influenced so many in a positive way. As you know he is Daddy's hero, a combination of a sharp natural intelligence and knowledge with honesty, humility, drive and high morals, the kind of mix that makes you survive and automatically morally commits you to push and improve the world they inherited. So, which mold I fit the best, the shy, creative and compassionate giver, or the extrovert, passive and self indulgent receiver? None of the above, for good or for bad! I cannot be anything more or anything less than what I am the reason why I chose to do things my way.

I honestly cannot help but to have always judged both our parents as if they live in another planet, detached from contemporary living values and reality except when Daddy says and behaves like what he claimed to be, a free thinker not for sale. This is contrary to what we all experience in our daily existence. Most people cannot live up to those standards because they will be out of a job before a cat can wink his eyes. I know that, I had that experience working at Wal Mart in Daytona Beach when I was let go. If you are honest, you embarrass your supervisor, imagine! Same frame of mind was working when I dated Alejandra early on when she was my favorite girl-friend, at a time when the term meant just that, no touching allowed. So very different from what you see today in the social media.

CHAPTER

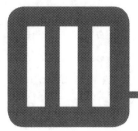

In my private world I always lived two different lives as a permanent bachelor since I left Alejandra's company behind as a kid, never to see or hear from her again. When I was gainfully employed reality was markedly and qualitatively different from what I found as soon as I returned to our parent's home where we lived with all the other permanent male bachelors until Mom died and Daddy remarried 2 years later. You girls were then living in Maryland where I was born. I moved in with Daniel, the talented architect brother who had earlier fled the Cuckoo's nest to design and build his own house when Daddy remarried. He had wanted to eventually get married and design/build his own huge family house like ours which he had also designed and build, but why wait, he wanted to become independent when Mom died. When Daniel left the family nest, somehow I felt the same insecurity and anxiety I experienced when Angell Jr. left to join the Navy. I immediately visualized in my mind the same negative signs of family problems that would follow thereafter. So we moved to Daniel's house where all 3 brothers shared each other's company . . . . but not for long. Soon after moving just 6 miles away from Daddy's house in Deltona where he lived alone with Suzi in a huge 7 bedroom house I felt an outcast and got involved in daily frequent reveries about life in Kensington Maryland where I was born while my platelets continue their descent to critical levels, still upset after being abused by Wal Mart.

One April the 6th. winterish springtime morning at Georgetown University Medical School hospital in Washington, DC I had started the protected, secure bubble life I am still in as I write these notes. My mother, as expected, enjoyed all the privileges and special considerations the wife of a faculty member was traditionally dispensed, so I was told. After a perfect delivery with no complications, I was soon released to our big home in Sonoma Road in Bethesda Maryland, almost a walking distance from Navy National Medical Center, Armed Forces Radiobiology Research Institute where Daddy would later on spend valuable time in research. We had a huge yard leading to a basement in the Rock Creek Palisades area. Little did the family and our huge dog Romeo know that eventually the creek would find her way into that most beautiful paneled basement where Daddy had his office and Romeo made his home. You girls were not born yet. All I remember is that life was all about Angell Jr when Daddy returned from work. Then Daniel you were born at same hospital, same results, same everything except that you were, like Angell Jr. a large 27 inches long baby when born.

I was too young to understand we were all living at the center of the world during the wars preceding the explosive Spring awakening that still rages in the Middle East, all fueled by the information technology. I was also too for Daddy to mold me like hid uncle influenced him with imaginary and real trips to planets, deep snorkeling waters where he swam and fish in the Atlantic Ocean under the blistering sun that matted his hair to the texture of a bleached rope. Dad would tell us how our Hispanic and Irish descendent families made it to the U.S. from Europe registered or not at Parris Island before the advent of the search tools in the I-net, if you can believe them. Angell Jr., also too young for the details, could absorb much more of the fiction. However, later on, as an adolescent I was able to corroborate by personal inspection the consistent accuracy of his descriptions and understand better Piscean fascination with the sea Which I also developed and enjoyed when snorkeling and fishing at the very same places he had with the company of Juanchito, youngest son of Santiago Bobonis, Daddy's first cousin and brother. The sandy beaches, the green coconuts hanging high from the tall, erect palm trees, the occasional Tsunami-like tides trying to flood the primitive Pinones resort areas, clam digging, oyster shells opening, crab hunting that eventually turned me into a fishing club life membership I still pay for. Angell Jr. and myself didn't have to have supper and then given a thick book to spend the early evenings reading—by the kerosene lamp—about the Marxist Revolution as seen by the Red Dean of Canterbury, England, the classic "The Soviet Power" like Daddy said he did. Instead, he would take us to his office inside the linear reactor at the Armed Forces Radiobiology Research Institute that got Angell Jr. thrilled. I couldn't care less.

I had also learned early to swim well, snorkel, and manage small canoes with the help of my cousin Juanchito but I always remained lonely, sad, and dejected but overtly smiling. Never did I have a fist fight with anyone.

I remember now how recently I felt something ominous was about to happen and felt a longing for Pinones and wanted to visit Puerto Rico again. I missed that deep water submerged canyon area near a wharf, 'El Ultimo Trolley', where sometimes, on week-ends, I used to accompany Juanchito and practice deep sea diving with the latest fishing gear equipment instead of the home-made pointed iron rod spear attached by its rounded end to a length of rubber from an old Firestone rubber inner-tube that Daddy used long time ago. How time changes. Later on in life Daddy confesses how much he regrets not having enough time during our early development to spend with us fishing or just daily after work informal sessions about the hierarchy of values where needs come ahead of conveniences, where the content of books or people deserve more attention than the dress or book cover, where axiological considerations always come ahead of physical satisfaction, etc. like his Uncle Agustin did after work. He did not have time but he made sure that weekends were for the family and Sunday mornings for church as we all occupied a whole bench at the Montellano Catholic Church.

By now you all must be getting bored again about my ramblings but I felt I had to get it out of my chest before I pass away any time soon. Before that time comes I really want to apologize to Daddy for his intrusions into what I then considered my private secret about getting treatment when I wanted to die. I hope he reads this and forgives me. I remember when he told us all how his tall, strong, balding uncle/hero, upon returning from work, empty lunch box in hand, . . . he would hug me and bring stability to my quotidian sad life along with Ana Luisa, his oldest daughter, who cared for Daddy and his baby needs as if he had been her own son. I remember with regret the times when I made an angry grimace when I knew he would ask me if I had taken my medications. He was hurt but wouldn't complain, I feel like an ass.

As you know, the other confusion about mother keeping her maiden name at Daddy's suggestion and his official ('de jure') degrading his last name to a middle initial 'O.', something he said that had 'de facto' already happened for a long time and caused a lot of problems to all of us after the terrorists' paranoia everywhere. How you finally managed to get it all straight to get your top secret clearances was an accomplishment, I didn't bother to do anything, for what? Dad was right to exalt the mother he never met and ignore the father that ignored him. That is the reason why he is so committed to provide all of us the things and answers he never got from his own parents. But he was diplomatically obsessive/compulsive about it, like we did not notice. ☺ But, come hell or high water, he was always there for us, no matter what. It must be very embarrassing anyone to have earned so many academic medals and distinctions and see nobody in your family during the ceremony to feel their pressing hand shake, feel their warm embrace around your neck or their gentle lips touching your reddened cheeks overcome by emotion. Instead, I was forever reminded that my only sister Virginia had all A's.: "She has always had A's in her school record, never a B." He always told us that this warning was often followed by having him learn the Spanish 28 letters of the alphabet with colored cards soon after he was able to sustain a stable erect position from crawling! He was able to read before he could walk! Cool! He tried the same approach with us boys and let Mommy handle you girls. This is why you always thought he had preferences for the boys who could get away with anything . . . . like what? He was always watching directly or indirectly through friends! We couldn't get away with any impropriety; his watching and protective eyes were always following us everywhere, anywhere as we grew up! If he had known the abuse Mrs. Santa Pinter had me suffer during my studies at Catholic primary school, all because I only spoke English, knowing Dad, he would have had her thrown out as a teacher. I guess Mommy suspected but Dad was very busy herding the prima donna faculty members into effectively reaching the freshman university students, that Mom didn't want to distract him with relative trivia. Was it trivia?

Remember, there was a house chock full of five kids, dogs, cats for Mom to look after and attend to all our needs in our household to be able to handle the 'Mrs. Santa Pinter effect'. But I survived it even though I was always day dreaming in the classroom when I attended classes, as if entangled with inhabitants from other planets in distant galaxies. But once back from school we boys roamed like stray cats all dozen acres of the University campus real estate looking for real and imaginary critters around, a round of tennis, or a deep in the faculty swimming pool and of course, holding hands with my beautiful Alexandra. That was life, who could ask for anything more . . .

As I mentioned before, Sundays was a different story taken up mostly by our church parish rituals and activities. Back at home from service I had the best of two world cosmogonies, the liberal theism of Dad and the conservative Orthodox Catholic line of our mother. I was becoming a moderate, a free thinker myself and somewhat of a conciliator in disputes with friends and family alike. Nobody paid attention to anything I ever had to say because I couldn't say it forcefully enough to draw attention to myself. The loud, controlling, macho style was more effective in impressing people, regardless of the message content. There was no room left for the soft spoken idealist activist, of the shy variety like yours truly. I didn't publish anything anywhere and if cut off mid sentence by those eager to be heard in their pronouncements, I didn't bother with finishing with the other half of the sentence or trying again, why should I?

How I miss those memorable High school years . . . . , swimming pool, music band, the tennis court, walking treks with the dog, playing with the deadly black widow colony our parents didn't know about . . . . no distractions from cell phones or I-pods.

But good things don't last long. Before you know it, the bright sunny days' perspective in the horizon starts fading away and becomes the new stark reality of the present . . . . as I wait for Godot. My world had already collapsed when we left the island and as a result, I lived in a trance and felt that I, too, had begun to die. Nothing really changed much thereafter as I tried to keep my disillusion carefully under wraps by trying to do things my way, challenging conventional operating procedures everyone else followed.

Unlike my other two brothers, I was not so eager or determined to enroll in the National Guard or reserves to earn a little money while I studied and thus become a little self-sufficient. I lacked that adventurous lust to travel and explore that most in our family had. Unlike most of you, I didn't have an honors registration at the university based on college entrance examination scores but I managed to get admitted into the university hotel administration program with Cornell University. By not getting involved, like my two other brothers, in military pursuits I felt was my way of not endorsing the continuous monopolistic capitalism ventures of the oil cartels.

I still miss Puerto Rico's mountain range paradise to this day more than 20 years ago, never to come back alive, especially now when I gaze way yonder from Florida at the southern skies in clear starry nights, across Lake Louise, looking for the Scorpio constellation and the moon, harboring a death wish in my heart . . . one that likely torture or slowly kill Daddy. Why does he insist on saving me? Why spend all that money for tests and evaluations that come down to the same conclusion, lupus, liver disease, bone marrow depression, low platelet count, same diagnosis, same therapy and the same results. Seems like all clinical visits were scripted to end in a departing scene, "You are ok, for now." the nurse will say with a parting smile. But I knew better that there are problems you cannot ever solve, a broken heart and the death of your loved ones . . . . When will this agony come to an end? The more things change, the more they stay the same.

CHAPTER

Before I tell you about my planned last attempt to solve my problems with Alejandra, let me first tell you one additional recent problem that has really complicated life for all of us here in Deltona since we came to live here after Daddy's retirement. Have you not wondered why would anyone like Daddy continues that obsessive compulsion to spend our precious family time trying to explain crazy things like life, consciousness, language acquisition and processing, brain neuronal representations of information and their translation into both inner and reportable language, etc.? Why not better get another paid job or spend your unpaid time during retirement in sports and entertainment at the golf course or occasionally enjoying time at a bar with friends? Why does he keep up this compulsive drive searching for explanations about an invisible world he dreams about? Does his mind hallucinate? I never saw him taking drugs other than red wine 'sleeping pill' and his coffee addiction. Do all people with a hypothesized overabundant supply of gray matter go crazy? Or is this a form of wishful messianic ambitions to control our family minds or sharing some universal connectedness or something? His slow but unrelenting drive to analyze, scrutinize and forever search for a reason or explanation for anything and everything that moves, or not, is just plain crazy. Or maybe this was his 'drug' addiction to escape from continuous grieving pain? This is enough to drive anyone normal around him to experience or witness on a daily basis. If not, ask fussy Suzi, his elegant pretty wife, always moving around solving her own family's unemployment or health problems in perpetual motion along the fast track style of her existence. All of which makes one wonder about what proportion of Suzi doers and academic dreamers society needs for peaceful survival? Can our Volusia County drivers survive without Suzi-like auto mechanics . . . . ? No! Can they survive without Daddy-like experts in classical auto mechanics theory . . . ? Definitely yes! However, should people be free to choose their hobbies after retirement, like I did after health enforced 'retirement'? Some retired academics choose to be entertained, bar hopping, playing golf, stamp collecting, bed hopping, watching television, lawn landscaping, reading, cooking, playing music or travelling. But some choose to learn and share, like I chose to play an instrument, and fool around with music electronics in my spare moments as a hobby. I also closed my eyes and see myself leisurely fishing along the shiny waters of the Atlantic Ocean in Puerto Rico or St. John's River in Florida. To each his own, everyone will do things their own way, and why not? As long as you don't take away anything properly belonging to others, what could be wrong with marrying your computer in a joint search for invisible objects to be arbitrarily represented with letters, numbers or words so you can now play with them using also arbitrary and convenient logical rules of play? Should that healthy, conscious choice be considered a hobby or a psychopathological behavior sometimes termed 'sane psychoses'. Anyway, why should anyone be saved even from enjoyable psychic, indulgent self destruction . . . . ? Is that different when 're-Mom' Suzi reads, does civic work, writes well when inspired and tends to her flowers, curtains, ducks, egrets, dogs, cats, . . . and us? Our family has always enjoyed social participation in many civic organizations for a long time, Rotaries, Elks, Knights of Columbus and VFW; should that not be enough social communication? They also attend together two different churches to socialize. The problem is that one is considered an antisocial loner and the other is a social extrovert. Why worry because a formal education shyness is often confused with conceit and aloofness. Give Dad a glass of Pinot Noir or a shot of Haig and Haig Pinch and watch him relax and released from his inhibitions in the social group as he repeats same improvised corny German jokes as the yawning, un-interested rest wonders what the hell is he talking about. Anyway, if he gets carried away and briefly exceeds that limited liquor quota of liver poison, he will return it back to mother earth in convulsive, uncontrollable bouts of oral greenish recursive jet ejections. Remember when Suzi would drive their new Nissan Altima back home with his head hanging outside the opened car window to inhale fresh air and resuscitate. And still, this crazy old man would, before going to bed, dutifully check his computer for exchanges, comments or replies from the Mega International, Omega, Prometheus, Mind and Brain, WedConscious, Ispenet or other 'one in a million' HiQ listings he participates or monitors, all worldwide groups specializing in all aspects of brain dynamics. Many a times he fell asleep in front of the computer monitor. Other sober times, before falling asleep, he gave thanks to his virtual God of choice for all blessings conferred upon him, family and neighbors, nation and earth . . . Not surprisingly; he said he had to re-read the last few communications again the next day.

What I barely understood from his mania was his insistence on telling his audience was not to waste their precious time on radical exclusive extreme mathematical logic abstractions or mystical religious pronouncements but to spend more time with solving real-time problems here on earth before engaging into intergalactic other world's mystical issues. That what we need was to reconcile what each extreme had to offer in a unified account. In my opinion, that meant to bring those conjectures and speculations to bear more directly into human health, psychic happiness and social conviviality, i.e., pay more attention to the real needs of real people in their pursuit of an individualized, fitting biopsychosocial equilibrium, plain and simple. What this and other more complex considerations meant is beyond my understanding but I knew brain scans and DNA transcription were involved somehow. He enjoyed his dream world and I was trying to enjoy mine, that's free choice, that's freedom. That may explain why these last few months when my health conditions had continued to deteriorate, I dressed up in the latest sport fashion shirt-pants combination only to stay home and spend hours dreaming about catching salmon or some other big fish with the latest fishing gear I had ordered and still sitting in my room at Daniel's house. I remember when Ken Collins, who still hangs around here, kept asking me where would I park my yatch in the house after I paid the last installment! I couldn't afford a bat with tall sails but I can dream about owning and riding one? What is the difference between one reality and the other, isn't all of human knowledge relational? As, what is cold without heat, light without dark or good without evil? Or as they say, perhaps conscious free will and unconscious determinism, structural/functional order and random chaos, sense phenomenal and ESP virtual reality, are simply different propositions about the same arguments of scientific logic? Look at your inert solid gold ring and confidently touch and sense the solidity with your fingers. Would you believe what science tells us all that, not only that a solid ring consists mainly of empty space! Not only that but also that inert objects, such as gold rings and rocks, consisting of particles whirling round each other trillions of times a second may be alive! It's like saying that inert objects, like plants, like ants or other animals move also even though we cannot see the motion with our naked eyes or even sophisticated instruments. If that is not confusing and crazy, I don't know what is! Likewise, as I have repeated so many times, we are ALL believers in some entity we may want to call God or something else, still the same thing. I mean, it all may be right, just "traveling the same circle in opposite directions." Because what is any God if not just a symbolic conceptualization of perfect order and harmony? History has recorded myriad conceptions of God since the dawn of civilization, from the monotheistic God of Judaism and the Trinitarian God of Christians to the non-theistic Buddhism. In fact, the characterization of the same conceptual God of order and perfection comes in all Jewish, Christian or Islamic flavors and yet vary so widely that there's no clear consensus on the definition of the exclusive God that different theologies claim, including materialistic 'atheism' belief in a strictly corporeal (material) world with no afterlife remnant. The classical believers believe God has an incorporeal (immaterial) existence, and that there's an afterlife reality or motion, like in the plants or the gold ring nobody has ever seen, heard, smelled or touched. As Daddy keeps repeating so many times, there is a real need to explain to the better informed computer youth why we hybridize our model of existential reality to incorporate both material and 'immaterial' aspects as being essentially a co-relative unit. This is another way of saying that "Life and consciousness represents seemingly invisible one side of the equation, the visible matter and measurable energy the other." This is why no one can deny that the current scientific paradigm is properly based on the belief that the world has an objective observer-independent existence, including the human species. But observers we are, only that our sense phenomenal experience as observers of ongoing objects and events depends on our brain, no brain, no reality. We build our understanding of its perceptual and conceptual aspects based on the known limitations of our human species to resolve the details of the invisible reality we cannot see or measure but intuition and common sense tells us it must be there. A big mystery, a pitiful state of affairs we all have to share. Same thing that happens in the science some have a blind faith in. Thank God I don't have to worry much about it. I have my own chosen cup of cake to let me carry on and through life, whatever it remains left for me. This is an example of what computer technology has given us younger generations, for good or for bad. I don't care . . .

CHAPTER

V

Believe it or not computer technology access to a worldwide audience has two competing roadways to information you either need or desire, is your own free conscious choice to decide as young adults still living with our parents and about to leave the nest by choice, not forced. Angell Jr. did, and so did Daniel and Nini. We all make decisions based on our mixed inherited and learned endowment. We are all sometimes unwilling creatures of circumstances but common to all of us healthy human beings is our natural drive to live and let live, be happy and make others sharing our turf also happy, and being socially accepted by others in convivial interaction with us. But we need to be alive, healthy and happy before we can reach out to others and share, in that order. This is what we have in common not only in our family but we also share with people we don't know outside the clan. But we also have special inner eyes and ears that are different and make you be yourself, like you are. We all live our lives our way if we can get away with it without pain to ourselves and others in our environmental midst. Some people, as antisocial and shy as we may project their personality to anyone within sight or speech range, we cannot live alone even when there is not an economic dependence mind set lurking behind. So we live with our wives, parents, children, partners or friends. So I chose my family as did most of you, nothing wrong with that, we are not 'mooching' as may seem on first sight. Every person is a world, an independent equation unraveling its contrived signature content as time passes. We all do things our way because there is no other way unless you wish to hang nailed to a post or cross in behalf of humanity, third parties or ultimately your own selfish self.

That is the reason Angell Jr. left the seemingly secure Cayey nest after high school and took flight never to return to the family fold until destiny had it that he really had no choice left but to let himself be trapped in our parents trick to come back to Deltona even before our house was completely finished.

And this is the same valid reason Nini flew out of the Cuckoo's nest and took flight to Maryland to continue studies and realize her dreams according to her individualized equation of life. Ditto for Daniel when he decided to invest in his own home and also leave the comfort and freedom he enjoyed in the Cuckoo's nest with our parents. In my case I inherited, like all of us did, from the same genetic pool and pretty much had equivalent learning environments, yet, when I was healthy, happy and liked by my friends and neighbors, I consciously chose to cast my future within the security, protection and love of our parents is because, I was welcome, to begin with, I felt comfortable and was not taking away anything that justifiably belonged to any of you, our parents or anyone's else to my knowledge. Yes, I knew that to the extent that you depend on others you also lose your freedom, but I could live with my conscience if I lived my way and nobody was hurt that I know of. It was an unexpected medical event untimely scheduled by circumstances beyond anyone's control to change that has hurt my family, but how could I have changed anything, all things considered. The only way I could think of was minimizing the high expensed of my medical care when I felt the outcome was written on the wall, the die was cast, nothing could reverse it, so why not live the remaining time my way . . . .

What no one in our immediate family can understand, myself sometimes included, is why the evolution of this complex pattern of events in my life was generally anticipated at such times when I was healthy, having fun with all my friends, the special one—Alejandra—included, during the Miguel Melendez Munoz High School years. It all started when Angell Jr. left the nest as I mentioned earlier. I knew that, sooner or later, we would all leave Puerto Rico, never to return, me at least . . . . now as I wait for that moment of death and transfiguration.

It now feels, as I look back in time, like the last chapter of a never ending space flight trail away from Puerto Rico, across the crystalline blue Atlantic Ocean waters, our reduced family finally arrived at India Boulevard in Deltona, Florida. Until I could find a job, I had plenty of time to reminisce the good and old times in those high mountains in Central Puerto Rico. Reconsidering now, my saga may have really started when Alejandra called me on the phone that unforgetful afternoon to let me know it would be in both our best interests to better discontinue our committed relationship, fully endorsed and approved by both our sides of the family. I couldn't believe I was listening to that as I audibly sobbed for even my sister outside my room door to hear. Was that ending the beginning of the impending end I am waiting for? What would now I do without her? I knew she couldn't wait to graduate High School and leave what she dubbed "her suffocating, controlling Chilean family". I knew and we both had discussed and considered different plans for that important moment. What now about her future, what about mine! I suspected she was perhaps looking forward, or maybe already found, to find that controlling macho Hispanic type, the 'Sharia law' Muslim-like variety to settle down with in marriage. I was not the type, unfortunately, far from it. I am still at times reminded by some of you, who witnessed the 4th. of July spectacle of sound crashes that the raging fury display of flying objects hitting the walls inside my room that followed immediately after I crash hung up the phone. When I came out of the room the first person that saw the tears cascading down my reddened face and cheeks was you Barbie, remember that? Of course I could never match the explosive outburst Angell Jr. displayed when frustrated or angered about some trivia. That was the only compensatory response I was reflexly able to muster to counter the deeper sadness the unexpected news had triggered in my heart . . . , and still does to this day. But I promised myself that one of these days I would face her again, my calm/diplomatic style and properly relieve myself of any guilt for perhaps having raised expectations in her I couldn't realistically fulfill or any other intentional ill will to hide or deceive. As you know, I did that and now, having rationalized the whole situation, I have absolved myself from any deliberate deceit and apologize for any deficiency in my personality I have no control of. Now I am ready to leave this earth in peace. Boy that was some memorable encounter when we shook hands! To be honest, I would have rather embraced her and have both die there by the car she was about to board to drive away to this day. But I had to continue living . . . my way, the only way I knew that wouldn't hurt me more than I could tolerate before going insane. But I feel better now before I leave you all behind to continue with life. Please just stay together and help each other like God and nature meant it to be in behalf of the survival of our species, now and in all succeeding generations to come, . . . like Daddy always says . . .

CHAPTER

Dear family, you may be tired of my silly explanations about my crazy trip back to Puerto Rico in search of Alejandra because I just wanted to see her again before I died. What I never really told you was that I really loved her and will continue to do it after I pass into wherever we go to if anywhere at all because I really don't know. People from our younger generation cannot imagine is how a loner, antisocial person like me can read and learn from the computer and sheer lonely reflections loners have time for. I may not be talkative but I can see lots of thing my extrovert friends or acquaintances don't care to invest time on. It's their life in the fast track moving but getting nowhere, like life is an eternal ride on Disney World's roller coaster. But when inspired by Alejandra's memory of our best times together I lust on the good feeling experienced when I realized that my crazy last trip to the Caribbean Pearl four thousand miles south of Deltona, Florida just to see her is in reality that kind of sacrifice inherent to love and care for others than self. Both Alejandra and I had loved and cared for not only our pets but everyone we met in our long walks along the lonely university grounds off hours when all was calmed and quiet except for the chirping critters that amused us so much as we also loved each other in non-verbal silence and body language gestures. The existential sacrifices all concerned were willing to make in the conclusion of our young but committed relationship was not necessarily inconsistent with their intrinsic nobility and Christian values. I was as elated in my ecstasis then as I now was and remain grieving and hurting from our permanent separation thereafter.

I had it all planned such that your announced trip from Maryland to visit family here in Deltona, Florida for a weekend visit coincided with my return to Orlando,

Florida airport to pick you up and take you home. I was actually returning from a secret, unannounced trip I made to visit Alejandra in Puerto Rico and lovingly convince her to desist from her plans to leave me and her family to escape and become independent. I was hoping deep in my heart to bring good news about our rendezvous to surprise you at the airport. So before you arrived I left Florida and didn't tell anyone where I was going because I felt all of you would laugh at me for being so stupid and waste money on that silly romantic trip.

I left for San Juan International airport and, during the three hours travel time, could not resist laughing thinking at the many trips I had suffered before driving to climb those high mountains on the way to Cayey, Puerto Rico with a heating car engine from a leaky carburetor until a sudden stroke of genius made me turn the air conditioner on to extract the heat from the overheated engine even though the air flow was burning my face. The hot air returning from the cooling engine and coming out of the standard, classical AC vents really hot! Eureka, it had worked! It was a worthwhile effort to bargain need for safety against the convenience of cool air in a tropical summer. I even thought of patenting that idea. ☺ Then, when I arrived, I made sure I had rented a comfortable car at the airport, no more worries for me. I had started the memorial trek and was on the road on my way to a surprise I had not expected. Stay tuned.

I finally passed the Com Sat Satellite station on my right side of Interstate Road I shortly before I turned right on Barbosa Avenue and soon after that passing Montellano Urbanization on my left. I was thinking of the also memorable Montellano Catholic Church when my heart jolted when I saw Miguel Melendez Munoz High School at my left, just before having to turn right into Henry Barracks Campus of the state university. My heart was about to come out of my chest as I entered the horseshoe road and finally arrived and parked right in front of her family house. It was late in that summer afternoon after school classes. Alejandra happened to be outside her house at that time. I waved at her and she shyly waved back, looking down but I could read on her facial expressions she was nervous but happy to see me again, wondering if I had dropped from a helicopter or a satellite.

"Can I talk to you for a little while, I just came to pick something up and thought I stop and chat before I leave." I lied.

"Sure, why not. Let's take a little walk down campus, like in the good old times before." She almost murmured softly as she insecurely walked towards the not so hot engine car where I standing dumb not knowing what to say or do but to feel hopeful. She joined me and we, once again reenacted the same old walking trek while barely rotating our faces, looking around to see if her parents and other neighbors were looking. I was hoping her parents were looking for I knew they wanted her to marry me. The rest of the neighbors didn't care much one way or the other. I even saw the ducks trying to examine my car and picking at the tires with their beaks. Many old memories flashed back in quick succession as we reached the end of the horseshoe and turned right, passing in front of the university chancellor residence on our right. We passed in front of the building where Daddy used to have his office, facing the water fountain near Cuco, the big black bull sculpture, a cherished university symbol. There were hardly half a dozen people still meandering around as I walked, hands inside my pockets, alongside my sweetheart that was . . .

As we quietly and slowly strolled along the sloping hills behind the art museum near the other big, main entrance gate, where we so many times kissed when the resident professors were not looking, we looked around but nobody was there to greet or avoid.

I nervously took a deep breath and confess to my estranged sweetheart that I still loved her and wanted her to reconsider her plans of moving away from her parent's house back into what? I dared ask. The destination intended was an uncertain somewhere that worried me sick. It had been abundantly clear in Alejandra's mind, as I later on figured out, that perhaps love was necessary but not sufficient enough to sustain a continuous committed relationship, especially if we had to daily make an effort to reconcile our different personalities, something I always thought it comes naturally when you love someone, no matter what. But, I guess I was naïve and could not understand why she would want her 'freedom'?

"To do what?", I kept asking myself. 'In my book', as they say, there would never be any obstacles for her or any human being to pursue their ambitions and happiness, with or without my presence or consent because people are free to find their lasting happiness even if it would destroy me in the process. I really meant that and told her also before the separation as well. Was she expecting the standard macho response to keep the dependant woman under the Sharia-like conditions of 'happy enslavement'? Or maybe she had dreams of becoming 'somebody' that your typical macho man fears out of jealousy. Or perhaps she, out of revenge or lust, wanted to play out in the social environment, the macho equivalent of the free female spouse, a female sponsored Sharia law in reverse where both spouses share the same home but also somebody else's if the sexual hormonal conditions are propitious. I don't know. It could well be the excesses of a sorely needed and deserved woman liberation movement sweeping the planet.

Or maybe she properly felt as a free human being—that she was not or will not ever be ready to become—if she abandoned her fuzzy plans to escape into the 'intellectual wannabees dreaming role of becoming somebody' as the inevitable consequence of a proper committal to raise a family and the consequent result of being overwhelmed by so many expected family issues. However, Alejandra suggests that her remorse is due to my escapes into fantasy land, existential living mind set style where nobody is hurt, nobody cares and a robotic, non creative sensual life continues as their actors are more concerned with income, looks, pleasures and nobody seems to care about the serious aspects and demands of responsible living according to each one's intellectual and experiential resources. She perhaps thinks that she really loves me but also sacrificial and has no time and space to think otherwise, she rides in the fast track lane, the show must go on, ... the die is cast.

Well I may not be able to perform a complex brain surgery, help draft a constitution or plan a drone voyage to the moon, Mars or Pakistan but I attended college, learned music, paid my bills, abide by the laws, what else does she want from me? I believe I could have been, just as well, a loving, responsible provider with a smile to the loving Alejandra genius. Anything wrong with that way of living, what else is necessary, will anyone please tell me? Am I missing something here? Maybe the die was not cast necessarily. Either you float aimlessly like drift wood in a tide at the mercy of circumstances you consciously and willingly chose to ignore when you had the choice and resources to solve or you swim against the current and save yourself.

You all may be laughing in silence wondering why I did not act that abstract script in my own circumstantial reality? My answer to that is clear and simple,

I just don't know and feel like I am 'preaching in underwear', as they say. Our own curious father says nobody really knows why human beings exclusively are able to consciously formulate, evolve and nourish two drastically conflicting and antagonistic strategies for the survival of the species. One of them applies strictly for ongoing, immanent biopsychosocial day to day survival of the species, something that we share with other evolved subhuman species. The other strategy transcends and extends beyond the sensory world we measure, observe or try to explain logically and depends on unknown cosmic radiation effects affecting human lives and they are designed to counter humans known relative inferior capacity to survive in our hostile earth environment. It all sounds like a schizophrenia that simultaneously fuels both your conscious drive to stay alive by killing if needed to provide that need and at the same time it fuels also a co-existent but undeveloped potential in most humans to do the exact opposite under identical circumstances when the same human beings may instead consciously sacrifice their own lives by hanging from a tree or nailed to a cross, as the case may be, all in behalf a loved one, family, neighbor, community, country or the entire human species as recorded history accounts detail in the case of the prophets from all religions. These coexisting mental paradoxes are triggered into action by environmental contingencies, familiar or new unexpected ones. The difference in the prevailing response will depend on individualized circumstances of heredity and/or acquired learning in your environment where you grow up whether imposed or consciously chosen by a healthy individual. I don't know the details but even the dummy Johnny some people think I am, can understand the clear message and credible logic. Do you?

To continue with the saga of my 'silly' trip to Puerto Rico to see Alejandra, you can see how the computer technology we all so obsessively exploit in creating more options to achieve the worthy goal of a healthy, happy and convivial psychosocial environment has simultaneously made possible to discover the abuses of the irresponsible and generational rich and powerful ones whose visceral defensive reaction has created the economic chaos this rift has caused. Watch the news media and you will live in your own flesh the major problems triggered by the typical insecurity angst and rebellion qualia of the 60's generation amongst the young unemployed including you both and Daniel in your effort to timely pay your debts while, at the same time, being in dire need for valuable time to plan and resolve our own health and potential unemployment worries.

But my serious conversation with Alejandra was to no avail. She was determined to give in into what she thought was her destiny, with total but un-intended disregard for everything that would left behind and become past history, a broken promise, beautiful memories, home, pets and teary me.

Once again, I had relied on my recent careful handling of our past relationship before our family left for Florida. I felt there was nothing I could do to reverse the recent past events. I then got confused and also distracted away with my perambulations in search for an understanding of the future course my life would evolve into without her, which compassionately I had now spontaneously extended to include her. I really wanted the best of future outcomes for her, with me or without me.

I decided then to invite her for a car ride around to enjoy, as it were, my Da Vinci 'last meal' before my virtual crucifixion awaiting for my return to Deltona, Florida after picking you both at the Orlando, Florida airport.

"Did you notice anything in my destroyed ego demeanor when I met you girls at the airport?"

So, as we retraced our steps and walked back to my parked car by the horseshoe, Alejandra suggested some beautiful family restaurant way on top of the mountain along the 'Piquina' snaking curvy road to Salinas. She then proceeded to text a message to her parents about her trip to the restaurant, or so it seemed anyway. We then took off to the road.

As we traveled we could still see the town of Cayey below as the clouds slowly descended upon us and the sun was bidding goodbye as it slowly disappeared behind the Central range of graying mountains. I tried very hard to repress preformed tears ready to flow and embarrass me before I could turn my head away from her auscultation eyes looking at mine. I feigned having seen a flying object by pointing a finger to the object—that was not—to distract her attention. Meanwhile I kept all along again searching for answers for that mysterious self annihilating behavior of hers, my curiosity and love were actively searching for a soothing answer I could comfort with during my trip back to catch a flight departing from San Juan International airport to meet you girls at the Orlando, Florida International airport.

Upon arriving at some log cabin resort restaurant I kept examining the colonial, history laden pictures and murals by local artists that decorated the wooden log walls of the restaurant we were visiting. The place was your typical rustic, romantic abode; right on the mountain top where I could see both the South Atlantic Ocean wavelets as they traveled to the crystalline white sandy shores and, by turning my head to the south I could also see the warm Caribbean Sea waves as they traveled north and east from the Central American and Venezuelan latitudes. We were comfortably sitting in the very middle of both views. A real spectacle to distract me from facing what was really happening. I thought we were one of many guests for that long uneventful weekend. Then I noticed Alejandra responding with a hand wave to another one originating from a gentleman sitting at another table, possibly a relative or friend from the university. There was me, pitiful Johnny, a very antisocial, un-engaging TYPE A personality visiting with now quiet but extrovert and engaging Alejandra visiting at the inn with our own charged emotional baggage. I couldn't hold back from memory the unending trail of flashbacks about our dear walks along the campus making sudden stops to steal a kiss from each other as we dreamt and planned our future engagement and marriage before settling down in either Barrazas, Carolina or the Central Cayey mountains to raise our family. I also fancied about how Miss Kitty, my feral cat, would find her way back to whatever mountain we settled down after our marriage if we left Kitty back with you all. I would have to bring her along to live with us as she freely cavorts and climb trees around our own Caribbean log cabin before she would get exhausted and hungry, scratching at the cabin door, returning to beg for canned fish food and packaged kibble treats.

Finally, I felt I couldn't hold back my emotions, stood up and walk to the bar. I couldn't hold back my tears in front of the bar tender that lifted his eyes momentarily as he poured me some delicious Belgian Heineken beer inside my tall 12 ounce glass while I avoided direct eye contact by swinging my tall chair towards the breath taking starry cosmological skies. I was beginning to wonder also how I could possibly communicate with you girls at the airport or plane in case there was a delay in my return from Puerto Rico contingent upon the evolution of things with my sweetheart. I had to return Alejandra home safely before I take the Autopista road and return to the San Juan international airport to board a returning flight to meet you at Orlando International airport.

What if I convince her and both decided to elope and follow up on the plans to materialize our dreams into reality?

My heart was beating fast and I walked outside so I could savor my Heineken beer when I noticed some body language communication exchange between Alejandra and the lonely male guest sitting yonder, away from our table. My initial visceral, animalistic reflex was jealousy; maybe it was her contemporary boy friend that followed her up here. How would he know she was here? Or maybe that texting message was not really aimed at home after all? Who knows? Speculations . . .

He was a good looking 'pale face' like Alejandra, dressed with the latest custom fashion attire and looking like a prosperous 'go getter' type ambitious man, the gold digger woman go for? Envy followed in a natural sequence of events that evolve before reason takes over, if it ever will. In my case after I decide like an animal to seek revenge and act like the expected macho type I knew I was not. So I took several nervous seeps of beer before even thinking to plan my next step. Maybe there is nothing important happening, I rationalized.

The wind outside was beginning to sing like Daddy's old Charlie-Boy's howling dog sounds whenever any of our several cats meowed to be fed or let out.

"We all miss you dearly Charlie Boy, wherever you happen to be."

After a brief exchange of routine pleasantries with the bar tender, I courageously walked inside the building, asked Alejandra to introduce me to her male friend before we would have to leave.

"Remember, I still have to be able to catch my returning flight on time after the dangerous trip descending from these tall mountains."

I told her I had made no hotel reservations anywhere as I analytically watched every detail from the 'tell tale' unconscious facial expressions of her accompanying emotions. I knew all about her non verbalized spontaneous facial expression and body language and how they would be much more eloquent than any contrived, non spontaneous verbal utterance. She also knew me very well indeed and lowered her head and remained silent, maybe feeling guilty, feeling pity for my non macho control in handling the situation or all of the above and perhaps much more as yet undisclosed. It didn't matter, I had caught the answer and, thanks to God, reason, understanding and forgiveness was slowly taking hold of my nervous and unsteady self when I surprised myself praying for forbearance and control before she quietly and almost inaudibly, almost sobbing, said,

"I am sorry, I will always love you . . . God knows maybe someday far into the future . . . ."

That was my typical Alejandra alright. To my surprise, her boyfriend quietly witnessed the moving scenery, as if previously informed by my pretty but evanescing girlfriend, now becoming history.

The affluent looking gentleman had already, politely paid the bill ignoring my civil protestations. I left a tip equivalent to what I had consumed and he nodded in gentle approval. All three of us walked outside to the gentleman's brand new blue Chevy Corvette I could have never afford.

I could not almost contain my tears again! Damn, what a curse to erupt my inner feelings like a volcano without a control, I protested to myself. I didn't care, she was used to this embarrassing non macho, sorry spectacle. I hugged her, put my arm around her shoulder and walked her to the rider's side of the fancy monumental car whereupon I opened the door wide for her, as her boyfriend silently observed from the driver's side. I could feel with my finger the cloth texture of a familiar fashion white blouse covering her blue jeans. Of course, it was the unforgettable combination I was attracted to when I first met her after they arrived into our neighborhood from the Chilean Andes slopes. That couldn't have been planned because she was taken by surprise when I unexpectedly showed up at her house today but then . . . . , that texting message must have done it. Oh well, life continues. Off to the airport and then to Orlando International Airport, I hope d I had not missed my flight.

I couldn't get Alejandra off my mind during my subsequent driving to San Juan International or flying to Florida's Orlando International airport. Once inside the economy flight, this is how I had wanted things to happen. I was sitting near the window, viewing the graying skies finally turning pitch black. I closed my eyes and dreamt away my version of what could have happened at the resort, at the top of the mountain:

We dined together, sipped red Cabernet Sauvignon from the Chilean vineyards as I watched every muscle of expression on her face as she knew I would be doing, trying to read what's in her subconscious mind before she told me. She was beautiful to my biased eyes and nervous as usual. Several naturally curving light brown hairs were cascading down to her artificially darkened eyebrows covering the also natural signs of her frontal fissures. We shared a few trivial recent short stories before eventually turning nervously to each other as if pleading for emotional comfort. Almost as if a genuine first sight romance had been reborn from still burning ashes.

I opened up little by little, at every moment praying that my calm, slow and good mannered views on things would not be misconstrued as if preaching and criticizing her extrovert, vivacious, almost flirty behavior she knew I did not approve of but suffered in silent consent. This was her standard misconception of viewing me, the typical shy, introvert loner always riding up in a tall high horse, ready to pass judgments on her nervous demeanor and past experiences. I knew, I would be the last person to make judgments on people and their circumstances imposed on them by nature ot their growing environment.

As always, I always felt guilt and regretted passing up a typical friendly conversation at a bar, bragging about money, women, leisure trips, cruises. I'd rather listen, enjoy talk about computers, fishing, hunting, gambling games, or look at pretty girls sitting across the table.

I kept trying real hard to project into Alejandra my premonition of seeing her struggling, for what would likely evolve into unbearable days of grief and suffering dictated by her anticipated nomadic, gypsy like search for a well deserved stable environments of family, friends, church services, trips to the movies, all happening after coming home from eight busy working hours of creative or entertaining job.

She could always become the creative protagonist of that wisdom she is obviously capable of, there is no impediment I can think of. She could share them by her own special exemplary life story of love and compassion.

But she was not really listening to me and I was not sure this attention deficit was intentional. Anyway it was time for me to stop preaching and start listening to her familiar side of the story.

After realizing she was not really telling me anything I had not heard robotically repeated, I waited patiently and then suggested a walk outside. I was not making my point across what nature and circumstances imposed as a barrier. Why God?, I asked in silence.

She moved closer to me and took my hand into hers and gently squeezed it. That quiet sojourn atop the graying mountain slope landscape venture was a respite from Alejandra's heart-rending subconscious script. How sad, I complained to my God; why do you do that to her . . . . and to me? She projected a long look that could have reached outer space in search of something unknown. I also searched in vain for any sign of something . . . desperately looking in vain for anything, any miracle arriving from anywhere in high heavens to reach and change destiny.

I took her hand and raised it to my lips as she inclined her head to rest it on my broad shoulders. We were both synchronized on the beautiful artisans work adorning the rustic log cabin wall space above the chimney. She stood up, held my held my hand and we danced on the wooden dancing platform by the bar as I held her tight to my chest when she cried and walked to the blue Chevy Corvette. I followed her and opened the car door for her. She was teary and hesitant and Alejandra was finally able to kiss me goodbye. I watched her car speed away into the paved road heading back to the Henry Barracks university campus where I prayed would be her final abode of health, happiness and social acceptance if she only listens to her loving parents. Goodbye Love . . . .

End

The unexpected change from the 'ideal' high mountain range scenario to the just as beautiful 'real' scenario of flat Central Florida where all 'white elephants come to die' as the saying goes, was radically different. He could not handle the realities attending the radically different lifestyle priorities from the 'ideal' yesterdays of growing up with his mother Judy, an Irish immigrant herself from

County Mayo, Ireland, now dying from a terminal cancer, and the shock both encountered of adjusting to the radically different lifestyle priorities of the 'real' multiple cultural backgrounds converging in Central Florida as briefly illustrated below for Judy . . .

"An Irish Senior Woman In Modern Florida"

(Hepta (7) syllable rhyme)

That would have certainly been
Her last orchid of summer,
That lovely Judith has seen.
All her lovely companions,
Bushes, roses, evergreens,
Dogs, cats, birds, snakes or stallions
No other Irish can dream,
In Belfast, Mayo, Dublin,
Where Thomas Moore, Mickey Finn
Would rather play with Goblins
Or Leprechauns than stay thin
Like the rest of Floridians
Stick together like Indians,
Sweat the hot sun but stay clean,
Then fight traffic jams for hours
Irish temper controlled, not mean.
Ireland always in her dreams
Where lovely memories, flowers,
Friends, are fast fading or gone.
She barely breath or have fun
Praying "Oh God ease my pain,
I don't want to be alone,
As I join those who have flown
Before, soon I will follow,
Ireland and Florida gone,
Leaving my husband alone
When all old friendships decay,
His clumsy shyness forlorn
His shiny tears will cascade
Down his reddened face away.
Who would inhabit alone,
This bleak modern world for long?

End of Book

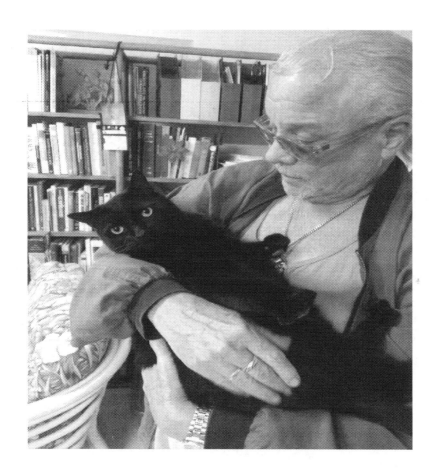

Chevy Boy in Deltona, Florida